PRAISE FOR

Touching the Light

"With the emergence of all the vast and new knowledge about energetic medicine, Touching the Light is the must have book for understanding home, health, and healing. It is a must read for anyone everywhere in every aspect of the field of health."

—DANNION BRINKLEY, New York Times *bestseller, author of* Saved by the Light *and* Secrets of the Light

"As a practicing gyn-oncologist, I have observed that western medicine cannot explain the phenomena of placebo effects and spontaneous remissions. It virtually ignores a host of potentially useful therapies such as homeopathy and energy medicine that do not fit its paradigm of cause and effect. With her unique ability to communicate with her non-ascended Masters, Dr. Blackburn-Losey has written the definitive comprehensive text that explains these phenomena at a level of understanding not yet known to the majority of humanity. I highly recommend this book as required reading to all those interested in the evolution of integrative medicine."

—MATTHEW BURRELL, MD

"In her riveting new book, Dr. Meg shares with her readers specific how-tos on developing your skills as a healer. In addition, she shares information about her personal experiences and how she learned to trust that what was happening to her was real. Thank you Dr. Meg for the courage to share your story and teaching the rest of us by your example to 'sit back and enjoy the ride!'"

—MARILU SCHMIER, author of Waiting for Weston: A Mother's Story about Raising a Multidimensional Child

"Merely reading the table of contents for Dr. Meg Blackburn Losey's new book will change your life for the better. Then, if you jump into the rest of her book, I'm sure you'll walk out at the end with a new kind of degree in Divine Sciences. In fact, much of what she offers here will have to become part of our regular education in the coming years if we are to advance as humanity from a body-centric intellectual race into the spirit-centered intuitive one we are destined to be. Hats off, once again, to Dr. Meg for mapping out for us a seldom charted territory of our spiritual development that we urgently need to understand. Pick up her book and pick a chapter like the one on what it takes to be a good healer, or about your etheric anatomy, or the chapter that addresses what no one wants to talk about, or the one on the healing session, and you'll find that any one of them is worth buying the whole book!"

—MICHAEL J. TAMURA, world-renowned spiritual teacher, clairvoyant visionary, pioneer of psychic and healing development, and award-winning author of You are the Answer: Discovering and Fulfilling Your Soul's Purpose

"This is a must read for everyone, and especially for those who are looking for alternatives to the confines of conventional medicine and Big Pharma."

—BOB FRISSELL, Flower of Life facilitator and author of Nothing In This Book Is True, But It's Exactly How Things Are

TOUCHING THE LIGHT

WHAT MIRACLES ARE MADE OF

HEALING BODY, MIND, AND SPIRIT BY MERGING WITH GOD CONSCIOUSNESS

Meg Blackburn Losey, Ph.D.

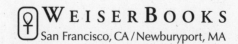
WEISERBOOKS
San Francisco, CA / Newburyport, MA

First published in 2011 by Weiser Books, an imprint of
Red Wheel/Weiser, LLC

With offices at:
665 Third Street, Suite 400
San Francisco, CA 94107
www.redwheelweiser.com

ISBN: 978-1-57863-462-0

LIBRARY OF CONGRESS CATALOGING-IN-PUBLICATION DATA available upon request

Cover design by www.levanfisherdesign.com/Barbara Fisher
Cover photograph © Velora
Interior by Maureen Forys, Happenstance Type-O-Rama

Printed in the United States of America
MAL

10 9 8 7 6 5 4 3 2 1

The paper used in this publication meets the minimum requirements of the American National
Standard for Information Sciences—Permanence of Paper for Printed Library Materials Z39.48-
1992 (R1997).

To all of the dedicated men and women of science who search diligently for cures to our ailments:

Look farther, try harder, and consider that which you can't prove.

The answers are not in front of you; they are within you and around

you. Touch beyond what you can measure and reach into the Light.

It is there you will find the holy grail of healing.

Medicine comes in all forms. It begins with a heart that is open to healing and is carried flawlessly by the emotions, where it is distributed throughout the body. It becomes first part of the energy field, then of the consciousness, moving through the body, communicating healing, and finally, culminating in the realization of the mind.

When we become out of balance with the field of creation, we begin to decay. We are no longer coordinated with the flow of creation and it begins to wall us off, compacting, even encapsulating energy around our weakest areas until we become sick or dysfunctional and our illness, our dysfunction, continues to deteriorate as blossoming doom. Decay becomes disease and our ultimate consumption from life to nothingness. If we do not become back in tune, in alignment with all of creation, it will consume us until there is nothing left.

It is the spirit that drives all healing. Everything else is merely a Band-Aid that we can see, touch, smell, or believe because it is something we think we can understand.

—MEG LOSEY

CONTENTS

LIST OF EXERCISES

ACKNOWLEDGMENTS

My heart to every one of my students, who have challenged me, required me to stretch, to expand, and to conceive of the endless possibilities that are available to each of us. Thank you for your interest and, yes, even your endless questions. They have been priceless. Without you I wouldn't have much to do, and I love you each and every one.

Endless thanks to my two models and wonderful friends Julia (Jewls) Hanson and Todd Andrychuck, who answered my call for sweet assistance and helped me get together the endless photographs that I needed so that the readers could really understand this work.

Many thanks to my friend Joseph Crane for giving me permission to use his long distance exercise in my classes all these years, and particularly in this book. It is a huge help in the leap of understanding just how far our healing senses can see.

Books by no means create themselves. Writing them is only the beginning. After that they come alive with the help of many people. To everyone at Red Wheel Weiser who had a hand in the birth of this baby, you always make me look so good! I thank you with all the gratitude in the world.

To my agent, Devra Ann Jacobs, thank you for believing in me all these years even before anyone knew who I was.

And to David.

AUTHOR'S NOTE

The health suggestions and recommendations in this book are based on the training, research, and personal experiences of the author. Because each person and situation is unique, the author and publisher encourage the reader to check with her holistic physician or other health professional before using any procedure outlined in this book. It is a sign of wisdom to seek a second or third opinion. Neither the author nor the publisher is responsible for any adverse consequences resulting from a change in diet or from the use of any other suggestions in this book.

INTRODUCTION

Alternative healing has existed literally for millennia. Evidence of poultices, herbs, and other remedies is found in archeological sites that are hundreds and thousands of years old. Traditional Chinese medicine uses many alternative processes for healing that include acupuncture, herbs, and energy to name a few. Medicine men and women continue to exist in tribes of indigenous people where they hold the utmost respect. These people are visionaries, shamans, and herbalists, and they often are gifted people who see the world in ways that we can only dream of. Over time, many significant people have come forward, offering new and different healing modalities such as Reiki, Theta Healing, EMF Balancing, Herbology, Homeopathy, and other modalities such as the healing methods that Barbara Brenan teaches in Hands of Light. Some of the new methods have proven to be quite effective, as are others that have ancient roots. Most methods offer, at the very least, the possibility that healing has answers that go beyond our current understanding.

If anyone had asked me years ago if I would be a healer, I would have laughed loudly, denying the possibility of such an idea. I would have been wrong. Really wrong, as I later found out.

My experiences in healing and the Etheric began almost accidentally; of course, we realize that there are never any accidents, don't we? My life had fallen apart over a period of about two weeks. Everything that I believed to be my base, including my accomplishments and my value system, came crashing down in every aspect of my life. Nothing that I believed in was true anymore. I was raw, really raw, and as I looked around one morning, I realized that something about how I was going about life had to change or I wasn't going to survive. So I said aloud to no one in particular because the room was empty except for me, "Whoever I am, whatever this is, *I accept.*" I have said many times since that moment that there are no more powerful words than those two because what happened next was the beginning of a mind-blowing series of events that continues years later and that has changed my life beyond words.

First of all, everyone who did not truthfully fit in my life, along with all of the illusions that I had about them and myself, fell away. I began to see how destructive some of the relationships in my life were. I saw how trying to please people who really didn't care took my attention away from what I really wanted. Many of the people in my life were using me for their own purposes, and in my eagerness to belong, to prove myself worthy, I had let them. I saw how my personal values were tools for my own destruction because they really weren't my values after all. Instead, my value system had become a parroting of the values and expectations of the people who had raised me, taught me, and mentored me during the course of my life. I had no clue who I was or what I wanted my life to look like, because I had tried so hard to fit in, to belong, to not feel so alone, that I had lost track of my own feelings and desires.

After my declaration of freedom, so to speak, I began to understand how profound the changes were that were happening in my life. Not only did people who were destructive to me fall away, never to be heard from again, new people began to appear almost daily who had different, more open and positive, outlooks. And I loved that.

In an effort to widen my growing positive circle of friends, I began going to a group that met weekly not too far from where I lived. There, many people gathered who were of a "new age" perspective. Being unfamiliar with such concepts and perceptions, I relished the freedom that I found there as I began, shyly at first, to state some of the intuitions that I had had, some of the things that I somehow just knew, and even my perceptions about others, which turned out to be more than just accurate; often they were prophetic.

As the weeks went by, I found that there was more depth to me than I could ever have realized in the life I had been leading before. I had real gifts, and I had withheld them for years because of the fear of being different, laughed at, or even admonished. I remember as a child talking about some of my experiences and how I was told that what I was experiencing wasn't and couldn't be real. In the Catholic school I attended, I was chastised and told that only *real* saints had the visions and the knowing that I had. I was just a kid. How could I know and see the things that I did? I was told my experiences were not real. I learned that I didn't deserve my own gifts because they were reserved only for those the church recognized as saints and miracle workers. I slowly learned to keep my experiences to myself, but even as I learned to maintain silence, those teachings never felt like the truth. When I asked questions or made statements that challenged what we were being taught, I was put right back in my seat in a hurry and admonished in front of everyone. They didn't understand that I comprehended the meaning of holy far beyond their idea of what holy must look like. Even as a child I had found a place inside of me that was vast and limitless in its possibilities. I also realized somehow that it was from my heart that all good things came. Soon though, I realized that secrets could be kept and my natural abilities were something to be hidden. As a result, I began to lose confidence and to feel insignificant, different, and apart from everyone else. It took over half of my life to realize that what I had been taught was wrong.

As I began to re-open myself to my natural abilities, strange things began to happen. At least, at the time they seemed strange. I started to feel as if someone was trying to talk through me. Not in a schizophrenic way, but honest to God, someone had something really important to say and they wanted to use me to say it. I fought it. Never was it my intention to be a channel or anything of the sort. Being a normal human being was hard enough. But it happened, and when it did, it was not only very real but also the true beginning of the expression of my gifts. I was unwittingly being cosmically launched.

One evening, a woman who had never been to the group before came to experience it. Being in kind of close quarters, the two of us found ourselves sandwiched together on the couch with one other person. As this woman inadvertently leaned on me, I couldn't help but see the inside of her right breast. I saw it as all light with two distinct dense areas. I silently realized that she had lumps in her breasts. Well, this was new. Seeing inside of people real time. Since my awareness was literally in there, I quietly allowed myself to experience the tissues, the densities, the differences, the energies, in fact, everything that her body was revealing to me.

Later in the evening as she was leaving, I don't know what possessed me, but I quietly went over and hugged her as a supportive gesture. As I did, I whispered in her ear, "There are two of them and they are benign." She looked up at me in shock. How did I know this? Who had told me? I had no answer for her and walked away with my own set of questions. What had just happened? What if I was wrong? How did I know this? Should I not have said anything?

After our meeting I found out that she had come to the group looking for some support while she awaited the outcome of her tissue biopsies. No one at the meeting had been told about her situation because she didn't want the attention. The following week I learned from our hostess, a good friend of the woman, that she had called with her biopsy results and that what I had told her was *exactly* what her medical tests had shown right down to the placement, size, and benign nature of the densities. I wasn't sure if I was shocked or relieved. Neither, I decided; it just was.

Another night, there was a young man in the group who was on a list for a kidney transplant. He was a juvenile diabetic and his kidneys were shutting down. Daily dialysis was keeping him alive. He was looking sicker and sicker each week, and I was very concerned about him. I liked him a lot. He was a very brave and humble person who was able to laugh at his situation and never asked for pity.

I had been channeling that night and afterwards my awareness remained very open as often happened. My young friend said something to me about his health, and all of a sudden, "we" began to read his body aloud, system after system, as if he were having an Etheric MRI. The information refined down to the fact that an adjustment could be made to the mixture that was being used for his dialysis that would give him more effective dialysis and that there were certain things that he could use to supplement his body to aid with the issues it was having. The experience was very much like I imagine people had with Edgar Cayce's readings and the cures he often came up with in his trance-like states. I was in awe, as was everyone in the room. I had no idea what I had just told him.

The next day my friend went to dialysis and suggested the changes that he had been given the night before. Amazingly, not only did the nurses apply the changes, he had spectacular results with his dialysis! He never told anyone where he got the information, just suggested from a lifetime of experience that maybe they would be better off changing a few things in his treatment.

As I began to channel more and more clearly, I realized that something strange was happening in and around my body. Energy was flowing as if rivers of clarity had awakened within my body. I felt as if I had been plugged into a naturally occurring energy conduit. The problem was that I couldn't find the release button to discharge all of the energy that was building up in me.

I was frustrated beyond words as, day after day, I was more charged. The feeling became so uncomfortable that I felt as if I would explode. Out of desperation, I got up out of my chair one morning and turned on some music . . . and I began to move. . . . I focused on my hands, because that was where the energy was most intense. As I concentrated on the energy in my hands, it grew, creating a field of warm, sometimes even hot, energy in the space between my hands. I moved my whole body with the music, slowly, rhythmically, concentrating on nothing but what was happening between my hands. As I moved with the music, the energy that had grown between my hands began to change. It became warmer, cooler, larger, smaller, and more intense, light in its feeling, and as my hands changed in sensation, so did my entire body. Every morning I repeated the process, following the energy instead of trying to command it. As I did, I felt calmer, more centered, sharper, more aware, focused, and completely out of my thinking self. I was on to something. I began to recognize that certain movements changed how the energy felt in my body and that I could adjust how that energy felt with tiny little movements.

As one morning after another went by, my awareness became sharper and the energy in my body flowed more freely, but I didn't know what to do with it. Every morning I began to say aloud, (no, the truth is, I *begged* . . .), "someone show me what to do!"

One morning as I raised my hands above my head and then lowered them outward, away from my body, I actually saw the energy arc over my head in a spectrum of color. A rainbow of color went from one hand over my head to the other hand. I was stunned. But then I became even more frustrated. I remember saying again, to no one in particular, "This is great, it's beautiful, but so what? *Now what?* What do I do with this? *Someone please show me!*"

What happened next was unbelievable. There in front of me, with no pomp or circumstance, materialized an extremely tall and absolutely gorgeous male being. His presence was a marriage between peace and power. Never had I felt such strength in gentleness. He wore a crimson robe and had dark endless eyes that went straight through his soul and right to the heart of the heavens. His hair was past his shoulders, long and brown with some slight wave to it. As he came into my visual field, I was understandably startled. All I knew in that moment was that there was a guy in my living room who came out of nowhere. I jumped straight up and backwards, shocked at my vision. And he disappeared.

What had I done? For weeks, alone in my journey, I had literally begged and pleaded with anyone who would listen to show me, hadn't I? What *had* I done? I quickly got back into my "space," as I had come to call it, and there he was, right where I had left him. I realized several years later as I recounted my story that he hadn't gone anywhere; I had. My startled emotion and following reaction had closed the door to my accessing this other reality.

Immediately upon my return to my greater senses, so to speak, my Etheric guest began to move in a way similar to the way I had been moving each morning. He was far more deliberate and graceful in his motion than I, and he stopped now and then to reveal to me what was happening to the energy he held.

What I realized from him that first day was that each little movement, each position of my hands, my body, and even what was in my heart and mind, had everything to do with what happened with the energy. So I began to mimic his every move. He never spoke a word, but somehow I knew everything he wanted me to know.

The motions of my body, my hands, and even my heart seemed to become a mergence of body, mind, and spirit. Gone were the circular thoughts in my head, gone was the stress of everyday life, and with the help of my new guide, I began to learn the secrets of creation. As I caught on to what I was being shown, the energies between my hands, in my body, and around me changed color, shape, even sound as my senses and awareness grew with my experiences. During the entire experience I never asked who, what, how . . . in fact, I asked nothing except to be shown more.

There came a time when I became generally frustrated because I did not know what to do with what I was learning. I felt like I had found a fantastic ride with no destination, and as a purpose-driven personality, it was difficult for me to just do whatever my guide did. I had no idea of the depth and the breadth of what he was showing me. Many years later I occasionally have yet another "aha" moment about those lessons.

I was getting very good at changing energy from one frequency or shape or color or sound to another. As I learned these things, the energy continued to build inside of me. I felt like a cosmic bomb that was ready to explode any minute. The intensity became painful at times and was overwhelming, to say the least. Soon I began to express my impatience to my guide, and one day after going through our motions together, he was gone, and I was met by another being with a wizened old face and straggly hair that somehow melded into a beard that rested atop his quite portly belly.

My new guide showed me how to transform energy into mass, how energy comes together to form reality, and how consciousness affects that reality. He taught me how to merge my consciousness with the construct of reality to create change in the energy I was working with.

To make a long story short, I experienced a succession of what I now lovingly call Masters. I never asked their names. They never told me. It didn't matter. What mattered was what they were teaching me. All of their lessons were far beyond anything I had ever heard of, let alone experienced. The lessons at the time seemed fragmented and non-cohesive. As least that was how it seemed. Only later did I realize how much I had really learned.

I used only one restriction in my relationships with the Masters, and it was for my own protection. Every day that I accessed my higher awareness, I was adamant that I would accept only teachers and guides who were of the light, with the light, and within the light and that no one and nothing else was acceptable. I had become so open in consciousness, I felt that if the Masters could access me, then so could pretty much anyone or anything else, so I was very careful about who I invited into my world and into my body.

Eventually, the Masters began to put the fragments of their teachings together for me. I remember a day when I had on my mind two different people who were not well for different reasons. I was both curious and concerned about them. As I thought about them during moments of altered consciousness, the most amazing thing happened. First one and then the other of these people began to rotate holographically in circles in front of me, as if they were weightless images laid upon an invisible turntable. As I watched, their bodies rotated, and I could see inside each of them. I could see what energies were out of harmony, where their bodies were dysfunctional, and even how to transmute those dysfunctions back to normal harmonic frequencies; I saw how to "fix" the problems.

Whoa . . . wait a minute. This was huge. This was the thing that miracles were made of. Floating bodies? Transmuted energy fields? What the heck?

To my continued amazement, the lessons kept coming. From the experiences of the free-floating bodies came visions and lessons in different healing chambers.

The first chamber had no walls or ceiling and nothing in the space except what appeared to be a monolithic alabaster stone that was flat on top, much like an altar would be. Above the stone rotated a body, and within it I could see tiny little interactions happening within the organic parts of the body as well as within the intricate workings of the energy field both outside and inside that body.

Later the Masters and I worked in a chamber that had walls of crystal and floors of stone. The place had an Atlantean feel to it. I was conscious of the fact that other beings were standing in the background in that room. When I questioned this, I was told that they were "holding space." I understood that they were holding the intense energy within a circle of nearly unseen Masters. As I looked, I noticed a depression in the floor a little larger than the size and length of a person. I was shown that, as a person lay in the depression, arcs of light would come from either side of the depression, seemingly out of the floor, covering and bathing the body in full spectrums of light. It was, I was told, regeneration. Somehow the spectrums of light attuned the entire energy field of the subject.

It was explained to me that just by living our lives we are affected by our environments, our emotions, our biology, other people, places, and events; in fact, the list was endless. I learned that as we are affected by these things, our energy fields constantly change to be in tune with our experiences. Our bodies also can become disharmonic, ill, or so sick that we can die. I was shown that light, in its harmonic frequencies, is what we are all created of. We can be attuned like intricate musical instruments back to a finely functional state that is not only healthy but also happy in every imaginable way.

I was led through a series of different chambers in which I came to understand not only about energy and our bodies, but also how consciousness works, how all of creation is assembled and of what, how creation becomes mass and reality, how multiple dimensions are not only real, but how they interrelate and align. I learned too how we are the consciousness within the living One, able to direct and redirect reality as we desire it, and how we literally exist on every plane of reality in conjunction with our human lives. I learned about holographic reality, but I didn't understand that until much later. And I learned more . . . much, much more.

I remember one morning as I got into my space, I instantly found myself standing inside of a pyramid of light. It was as if the pyramid by its defined energy became the room. As I stood there, I realized first of all that this room was more ancient than any version of history we have. Secondly, I realized that I wasn't alone. Standing next to me was a wrinkled old Master who emanated extreme seriousness. He seemed to be all business but with a force of strength and balance that I had never before experienced. He felt as if he were a fixture in all time and that all of history had been built upon his back. He wore purple robes, and I sensed that on those robes were symbols in extraordinary numbers. Funny, I couldn't see them, but the information that they conveyed was becoming part of me.

As I stood there in awe, I also realized that I was watching this scene from about twenty feet away. Wait a minute. I was in the pyramid. I was watching me in the pyramid. And wait, I was also a human being watching me watching myself in the pyramid, and in the pyramid I was aware of my other two selves and then . . . The Master stepped into me. As I looked down, my arms were now his, flowing with long purple sleeves with living symbols cascading down them like a waterfall of knowledge. My hands looked ancient and I could feel him inside me, directing me patiently but firmly. I felt as if I had become the embodiment of all history. My hands spontaneously began to move, and I realized that a fourth me was on the table in front of "us." Oh. My. God! I had gone inter-dimensional, but somehow it was okay. Somehow I was learning to simply have experiences with the Masters without having a need to question or have expectations.

As my hands moved, the energy in our mutual body changed. The energy emanating from our collective hands changed frequencies as it moved over my other body, the one on the table. In that body, I could feel changes happening while still I witnessed all of this from afar.

Trying to keep up with all of my simultaneous realities began to remind me of that guy on the old *Ed Sullivan Show* who spun the plates—one, then another— until he had a whole field of them spinning at once without any of them falling and breaking. But somehow the whole experience was effortless.

The more I asked, the deeper we went, the Masters and I. My desire to learn from them was insatiable, and absorbing their teachings seemed effortless. I never asked who, what, where, when, or why, I simply trusted that what I was learning would all begin to make sense at some point. And oh how it did.

I tried to share my experiences with other people, but either they thought I had lost my mind, or, even if they wanted to believe me, I was unable to express what I was experiencing in terms they could understand.

In an effort to maintain my sanity during those times, I had a couple of friends of long standing who I used as reality checks.

My instructions to my friends were that if they ever saw me going too far down the rabbit hole to the point that I became unreasonable, seemed dysfunctional, or just seemed really crazy or unable to function in the 3-D world, I wanted them to tell me. I knew I could trust and believe them to help me stay safe.

My sense of reality was changing so fast it was difficult to separate my Etheric experiences from the third-dimensional world. They all began to blend together. I began to see overlapping realities. I saw people leaving colored trails of energy behind as they walked by. I saw beings from other realities crossing over or passing through our earthly reality. I saw spirits from the other side. I saw beings of every possible color and shape. It was as if all of my reality filters had gone on vacation and everything was happening all at once. In fact, I learned that it was.

Eventually, once I got over how cool it was to see everything simultaneously, I had to get realistic. I had way too much input and it was distracting. I began to state the intention that I only wanted to see or experience what was applicable or important to myself or to the person with whom I was interacting. I also had to make the statements that I needed to earn a living, to eat, to sleep, to have some semblance of a normal life. Once we erase our Etheric boundaries, we access multiple realities all of the time, and they us. Beyond the third dimension, many beings are made of light. They have never had physical bodies that require eating and sleeping or making a living.

I can remember being so exhausted from my attentiveness to the infinite that I finally stated that I needed three consecutive days and nights off because I needed to go to work. Literally, for three days and three nights it was silent. No one appeared. It was like a vacuum with none of the daily (and nightly) surreal activities taking place. I rested and took time to nurture myself, to get grounded, to do normal human stuff. After the third day, they picked up right where they left off in their teachings.

"How do you do that?" I asked, because they always unerringly began right where we had left off.

"Easy," they said. "There is no time or space here in our reality. It is you who interrupts the flow and you who returns to it."

Wow. So I didn't have to hurry up and learn everything in case they left. It was me who entered the knowledge; the knowledge didn't enter me. This was learning in an entirely new way. What I learned wasn't mental in nature at all; rather, it became part of my very being. Its concepts and details were so vast that I couldn't possibly comprehend the enormity of it all, and, honestly, I didn't try. The experiences I was having were, in many ways, indescribable, and yet there they were.

I also realized that I was having these experiences for reasons yet unknown to me. All I knew for sure was that having these experiences didn't mean that I was more gifted, smarter, or better than anyone else. I had simply requested to be shown and I had listened. My passion became to put what I was learning to good use.

I began to work with a few friends in the way the Masters worked with me. I worked with the energies in and around their bodies. I didn't charge a dime for my time and, in fact, honestly told my friends that I had no idea what I was doing but that working with others seemed to be the next logical step. I had plenty of volunteers, to say the least.

I set up a massage table so that I could move freely around a person. As I worked, my hands would move as if they had been pushed into a new position. Often different Masters would "step in" to assist me. I became accustomed to the feeling of "us," whoever they and me combined were. Believe it or not, it became perfectly normal for me to look down and see someone else's hands and arms, their clothing, and still be aware of the me in that combination.

Later, other beings that were obviously from different planes of reality began to appear. I quickly learned that each person I worked on had a unique set of connections to beings of other realities. I used to joke and say, "Gee, that isn't one of mine!"

I saw guides, deceased relatives, angels, even extra-terrestrials as well as a variety of other beings come and go. I began to recognize many of these Etheric assistants and also became aware that sometimes they just came because they were curious about what I was doing. Okay with me; maybe we would all learn something.

As I became more confident with what I had learned, I began to see how the lessons could apply to everyday life. During the first year or so, I worked without charge with my friends; they sent other friends, who sent others, family members and more. Part of our agreement was that I would follow up with them after the work. So a day or two after each session, I called my clients and talked with them at length about what they experienced after their sessions with me. I began to see definite patterns of cause and effect. Those calls proved to be invaluable as I realized that the body tells a cohesive story when the information gained from all layers of energy is put together. We can interpret from the energy field what that person is experiencing in his or her life. Incredible.

I also began to see some pretty miraculous results. Tumors went away and didn't come back. Congenital defects no longer existed; lives changed direction; there seemed to be no restrictions on the possible outcomes as energy and harmonics were adjusted, attuned, and retuned.

A friend from our group who was an emergency room technician called me one morning and said that her daughter, who had a congenital heart defect, had tried to commit suicide. Her physician had just told her that she couldn't have children because it would be too great a risk of her own life. As a pre-school teacher with a lifelong desire to have children of her own, she was devastated. She had geared her entire college studies around rearing and teaching children. Now her dreams were devastated, and she didn't feel she had anything to live for. I told my friend to bring her daughter over and leave her with me. I talked with the girl as I worked within her energy field. I was passionate beyond words to save this life and to help her change her life to the degree I knew possible.

As I stood at her head, with my hands on either side of her face, I found myself entering her body. I looked up and realized that I was literally inside her heart. I was looking up right at her aortic valve. Mind you, I did not and still don't have any medical training. As I looked at the misshapen valve, I saw the possible reality that the valve was no longer malformed. As I looked, the valve changed until it appeared to be normal. Honestly, I didn't see this as any big deal, only an extension of what I had learned. Now I was seeing what was possible. During that session, I also saw that my young friend would successfully have children later on.

A week later, the doctor was blown away because her new tests did not show the congenital defect. Instead, they showed a normal heart and valves. He chalked it up to the fact that her medication must have worked. Yeah. Right. Medication doesn't change the shape of a malformed heart valve. Even *I* knew that. So did she and her family. What the doctor didn't know was that she hadn't taken the medication. The reason for the changes didn't and still doesn't matter. The fact is that it happened.

This year, my young friend is an ecstatic new mother with a healthy heart and a very successful pregnancy that resulted in a healthy baby girl. What an honor and a pleasure to have assisted in that journey!

My same friend has a son who was in the tree cutting business. A young entrepreneur, he had started his own business. While on a job cutting down some huge trees, he was seriously injured by a tree falling from a boom and pinning him against a truck. His pelvis was crushed.

His mother called me from the emergency room and told me what the x-rays showed. A quick glance from my newfound perspective showed me even further damage that the x-ray didn't show.

They came straight from the emergency room. He was on crutches and in extreme pain. I could see the fractures mending as I worked on them. As usual, I was in awe of what I witnessed. I told him and his mother that he was now fine, that the fractures were healing, and that he would be back on his feet very quickly. Within a week, he went for a return visit to the doctor and, oddly enough, was so well healed he was able to put down the crutches and never needed them again.

As this amazing new work and my experience with it grew in scope, people who had been afflicted in different ways no longer were. Life changed dramatically for many after our work; for me it was also changing. Unfortunately, my clients started seeing me as a miracle worker. I never meant for that to happen. They began to drive for days or fly from other states to be healed. My phone rang day and night. Flowers and gifts were left by my front door. This thing was getting much bigger than I, and there was no taking back what so many already knew. It was never my intention to be placed on a pedestal, only to share my gifts. Unfortunately, I quickly realized that the ensuing results of my healing efforts were making it impossible for many of my clients to see me any other way.

So many needful human beings came to me for help that I literally worked night and day, and eventually, I became exhausted and very sick. I developed stage three breast cancer seemingly out of nowhere. I was essentially told that I was as good as dead. The tumor was huge, the size of my fist, and quickly growing toward my chest wall.

Time to regroup, back up, and see what was going on. With all of the miraculous work that was happening under my hands, I didn't seem to be able to heal myself.

In a very profound moment, amidst mixed emotions and constant questions, the realization came to me that this illness was mine alone to deal with and that there were reasons for its occurrence that maybe I would never understand; I realized that I had to look at *me* deeply.

I had become lost in the intense acceptance by others of my gifts. Life became so different for me that I barely recognized it as mine anymore. I kept feeling that I wasn't giving enough, but at the same time, I was thinking, "What about me? Who had I become and who really cared as long as I "fixed *them*"? I cared. A lot.

I felt more alone than I ever had. I felt guilty simultaneously for not giving myself away and for giving myself away; I felt guilty for even questioning what had become of me and for not having set clearer boundaries from the very beginning. I thought I had, but who knew? How could I have predicted what was happening?

I began to unravel my emotions, to set the boundaries that I needed and to be even clearer with my clients about their part of the healing process. I helped them understand that *they* were responsible for whatever results they experienced because without *their* participation I couldn't make the changes they wanted. I am just a conduit. Aside from that, I am a human being who has needs, feelings, and emotions. So I began to set some boundaries to allow me to separate from everyone and to have some semblance of my own life in addition to sharing my gifts. And I am fine with that. So is everyone else. I did have surgery and had the cancer removed. It was too far along for me to do much else.

In an effort to help myself heal, I gathered together my closest friends whose healing abilities I respected and believed in. At a set time the day before my surgery, we all worked together to eradicate the tumor. I believed so deeply that we had healed the cancer that I was literally shocked to learn it was still present the next morning and that I would have to proceed with the surgery. I remember clearly saying that healing the cancer was mine to do. In doing so, I learned a great deal about myself as a human being. I also learned to see myself differently so that I wasn't so overwhelmed with my gifts. As of this writing that was nine years ago. I am still cancer free and life is amazing.

It is often difficult to get the message through to others that I am no different than they are. Any pedestal is too high for me. Everyone has gifts that they either acknowledge or don't. Either way is fine. There are no shoulds where I have learned to come from . . . only possibilities that are endless.

With practice, I have discovered how to communicate clearly about what I have learned and even found ways to teach these concepts that anyone can hear and apply. My students understand the concepts that I share with them, and often, they, too, experience having their hands placed for them or an occasional Master stepping in to help. As people make the conscious choice to step into this kind of healing work, not much happens that surprises me.

My students come from all walks of life, from housewives to physicians and lawyers. And every single student has taken home a different perspective of life in general and its possibilities.

In one class I taught in Atlanta, a good friend of mine who is an OB/GYN oncologist stood up to introduce himself as all my students do. At his request, I had worked with his sister who had breast cancer. She moved through healing from the initial cancer quite well and then one day I found that the cancer had metastasized into her brain. It had not yet shown up on her tests, but it was there.

She finally succumbed to the disease at exactly the moment she knew her brother was coming to see me for another event. Together, he, I, and everyone else in the room followed, through my Etheric vision, her transition from this life to the next; not a dry eye was to be found in the room. She was having a ball being out of her sick body and was singing an aria on her way out. The same aria was played at her memorial service later when the family gathered.

As he stood up in my class, instead of introducing himself first, my friend simply stated that I could read a body as well as any MRI, and he proceeded to tell the story of his sister and my involvement in her case.

Hearing his opinion of my gifts was a real wake-up call to the reality and depth of how people's lives were being affected by what I had learned. It also reminded me of what is possible if only we step beyond our belief systems and defensive modes into the unknown. This entire series of events and too many others to write about here are not just my awesome experiences. They have become the experiences of countless people who have both received and learned how to use their gifts in their own rights. All of this is very real and has been proven medically and otherwise over and over again throughout the years.

I want to make it clear that I am not a medical doctor. I am not trained in medicine. What little I know about "normal" medicine I have learned along the way as I have seen and encountered one situation after another, one body at a time. Part of my gift is to see inside the body on an almost subatomic level. I often see the inner working of the body on its most minute levels, and I have to honestly say that I don't always understand what I am seeing. I am okay with that. I can generally pull together enough words to convey what I am seeing.

I can be called a medical intuitive, an intuitive, a seer, whatever you decide, but to me the labels don't matter. All that matters are the possibilities and their applied outcomes. I am a conduit, not a miracle worker. I don't need or want credit for whatever happens in my hands. What I want people to know is that the real miracles come when those I touch believe with all their heart and soul that something can change, and it does because they let the change in.

It is my desire for you, the reader, to get outside your comfort zone, at least for the time it takes you to read this book, and imagine that maybe, just maybe, you are in control of your life and maybe, just maybe, whatever you desire is as simple as imagining it. And maybe, just maybe, healing is very much all about perception, energy, and our participation in our own journeys.

TOUCHING THE LIGHT

CHAPTER ONE

The Subtle Energy Fields and What Modern Medicine Does Not Consider

The stigma that conventional medicine has instilled against alternative, or complementary, medicine that it is quackery, doesn't work, and is ineffective, is arguably one of the greatest debates of all time. In many states and countries, alternative healing is embraced as both effective and acceptable, even complementary to modern, or allopathic, medicine.

Alternative Healing Unfairly Receives a Bad Reputation

Alternative healing has been given a bad rap for many reasons. It has taken on many forms, identities, and modalities over the course of time. Some have worked magnificently while others fell into the category of quackery, snake oils, and elixirs that did nothing but line the pockets of their inventors and practitioners. Like any subject, alternative healing has many faces and infinite perspectives.

One of the reasons alternative healing is difficult for many people to understand and the reason many people are afraid of it is that usually alternative healing comprises intangibles, and it is based upon the intuitions or experiences of others. Alternative healing incorporates supplements and methods of healing that are not generally accepted as proven in the allopathic world of so-called modern medicine, especially among the pharmaceutical companies who make billions of dollars with their products.

The truth is, we may not always know why something works, but if it does, the why and how shouldn't matter. In my many years of working with people and their challenges, I have found that the how and why just aren't what is important. What is important is that it works.

To me, proof isn't necessary when people who were very sick or challenged for some reason suddenly do an about face and are completely healed of whatever ailed them.

The Marriage of Conventional and Alternative Medicine Is a Match Made in Heaven

What we must also realize is that, quite often, alternative methods of healing can be utilized in a complementary way to so-called "normal medicine."

In my humble opinion and based upon literally thousands of hands-on and long distance sessions, there is nearly always room for the alternative to coincide with modern currently acceptable methods. Science is based on what is measurable and provable, and yet what I have experienced nearly every time I have been privileged to do this work is that what I see occur is neither.

Sacred Geometry: More Than Pretty Shapes

As the Masters taught me about consciousness, creation, and the relationships of both in conjunction to sacred geometry, it was a cosmic "aha!" for me. Suddenly I realized how prayers work, how miracles happen, and how we are part of everything and everything really is us. Really. Yet I couldn't prove it. I could only share my story, so a few years later I wrote my first book, *Pyramids of Light: Awakening to Multi-Dimensional Reality.* Truthfully, I went publically out on a long limb as I described the basic fabric of creation and how we are harmonically and indelibly linked within it all. I used geometric forms to tell much of my story, wondering if the world would laugh me into a small room where someone would throw away the key. Instead, almost exactly eight months after I published the book, the cover of *Science Magazine* had illustrations of geometric forms nearly identical to mine in an article discussing how scientists had just proven that in all of creation certain forms occur as matter and reality come to be.

I would never have known about it, but someone who had read my book emailed me a copy of the magazine cover. All I could think was, "Oh. My. God. This stuff I am experiencing is real. I *knew* it." Now I had a little proof. As time has moved on, science has occasionally caught up with my teachings. I celebrate

each and every time it happens because we are all of the same mind and sometimes we can witness that in a cohesive way.

Alternative Medicine, Pharmaceutical Companies, and the AMA

Too many times, the alternative has been shut down, hidden, or altogether obliterated in the name of science and medicine. That, to me, is just downright wrong.
For example, according to a terrific book on this subject called *The Politics of
Healing* by Daniel Haley, great damage has been done in the past by the American Medical Association (AMA) and other organizations of the medical world as
they literally squashed successful cures for cancer back in the 1930s that were
created by eminent doctors who took varied, and as yet untested and unproven,
turns in their research to real people who got better.

In the 1930s a man named Royal Raymond Rife invented a quartz crystal
light–refracting microscope through which he was literally able to see living frequencies. Instead of using, for instance, dried blood on a slide, he was able to view
blood in its living form under his special microscope.

Dr. Rife realized that he was viewing living diseases and that each different one went through several states of being. He realized that most diseases are
polymorphic; they move from, say, a bacteria to a virus to a fungus, and back to
bacteria. As he witnessed these transformations, Dr. Rife realized that each stage
of disease had a unique and specific frequency or set of frequencies. As he exper-
imented with these frequencies, he discovered that if he introduced the exact
opposite of the frequencies of the disease stage, the disease was obliterated. This
was a lot like having a Yin and introducing a Yang. The two parts negated each
other.

As his understanding of these processes grew, Dr. Rife began to utilize his
findings on terminal cancer patients. Patients who were so far along in their illness that their deaths were sometimes imminent.

And every single one of them recovered fully. All of them.

Dr. Rife had discovered the cure to essentially all disease. Imagine. When
news of his discoveries became public, the American Medical Association (AMA)
pressured Dr. Rife to share his technology because there was a huge amount of

money to be made. Like other researchers at the time, Dr. Rife wasn't interested in the financial gain or fame but in what his discovery could do for humanity. It wasn't long before the AMA destroyed Dr. Rife's lab, his notes, and most of his equipment, essentially ruining him and his work for any future use.

Many have tried to re-create Rife's technology and have come close but have not been able to exactly replicate his work. Part of the problem is that our current technology produces very specific tones and frequencies that do not fluctuate or waver. In the 1930s electronic machines were powered and modulated by glass tubes. Because the technology was more primitive, fluctuations in the sound, light, and vibrations occurred. It was in the imperfection of frequencies, the fluctuations, and the span in between frequencies, that the healing took place.

Rife's discoveries spoke loudly to us and the states of our perceived illnesses, and yet we do not fully hear his discoveries. There is little money to be made in wellness and huge sums being made through illnesses. Assessing living frequencies as they apply to the physical and energetic bodies will be the ultimate in curing all illness. Much like Dr. Leonard "Bones" McCoy in Star Trek, we will someday be able to wave a frequency assessment tool over and around a body to find exactly where the harmonic attunement is off and to correct the attunement toward a full cure.

The sad truth is that Rife's work was all destroyed because he would not get into profit sharing of his work with the AMA. Seriously. Dr. Rife was more interested in healing the sick than dollars and cents.

Others, including a man named Harry Hoxsey, came up with cures for cancer around the same time. Hoxsey observed that when his horse grazed in certain areas of a pasture, an ugly tumor growth on its body diminished. After many years of trial and error, Hoxsey came up with the ingredients from his field that obliterated cancer. His work was threatened and largely destroyed as well, but I do hear that a clinic based upon his research was opened in Mexico.

Another man named Gaston Naessens, who did anti-cancer blood research, began to understand how to read live blood samples and to cure cancer based upon what he found. He was only interested in the cure, never money or fame, but he was ostracized, raided, imprisoned, and destroyed by the medical powers-that-be.

Although Daniel Haley's assertions in the above stories have not been proven, they have a ring of a truth that is, on deep levels, hard to deny.

Currently, the pharmaceutical companies would have us believe that we can't live without their products, that we must be afflicted by certain diseases if we have certain symptoms. These same companies lobby to have all forms of alternative healings and supplements determined to be illegal or taken off the market. After all, they don't make money from alternatives. It is a very sad thing that the hard hitting corporate perception of reality is allowed to reign over more subtle truths.

When we moved to Tennessee for five years, there was only one doctor's office in our small town. A family of physicians ran it. When I walked in, I remember thinking how thoughtful that they had a new flat screen TV in the waiting room for their patients to pass the waiting time . . . until I realized that what was showing on the TV wasn't the daily soap or game show or even CNN news. Instead, they were advertising prescription drugs with a reminder to the patient to ask the doc if those drugs would help us while we were there. Once in the examination room, I noticed that the doctors had monthly digests of the latest drugs on their desks, all advertised by the pharmaceutical companies. I was encouraged on more than one occasion to try the drug of the month for this or that ailment. I remember telling the doc that the drugs were too new and that I imagined that within a year we would hear of a recall and the damage they had done. Sure enough, I was right. Frankly, I find this disgusting. We are not unhealthy to start with, but we can sure get that way in a hurry by believing the advertisements.

We can't watch a program on TV or listen to the radio, open a magazine, or participate in our world in general without drug ads in our faces. Many of my students who work or have worked in doctor's offices tell me that although it is illegal in their states, the pharmaceutical companies continue to reward doctors for prescribing their drugs. These rewards, according to a number of my students in areas where this is prevalent, apply especially in regards to children who are being blanket diagnosed with ADD and ADHD, bi-polar, and other horrendous labels they will have to live with forever. When I hear these things, they aren't told to me as gossip or even to convince me of anything. Mostly, the stories come from students who ask my opinion of the different situations they have witnessed. Needless to say, I am incensed when I hear these stories. Once upon a time, medications saved lives. Now I venture to say they run and ruin many lives. There is a time and a place for drugs, but not in the way they are being thrust upon an innocent public today.

Has anyone considered that maybe, just maybe, we are experiencing an evolution of awareness or changes in our energy fields that have caused us to physically begin to operate differently as human beings?

Case in point: autism. Without a doubt, autism is an epidemic and is completely misunderstood. A generation of our children is experiencing, in nearly epidemic proportions, a disease that has a wide spectrum of effects and symptoms. Why are the symptoms of autism so varied? Simple. It has everything to do with the subtle energy field. Since conventional medicine does not consider the subtle energy field at all, it has been missing the boat to effective cures and treatments for autistic children.

If the medical community were to look at autism from the perspective of subtle energy, they would find a completely different set of information from what is found in the physical realm. For many years, children's vaccines contained fillers such as mercury and thallium as additives. Mercury is conductive. It responds to temperature variations, it conducts energy, and it has been researched as a possible fuel for inter-stellar travel because of its efficiency and level of conductivity.

And what did our pharmaceutical companies and drug inventors do? They used these elements as fillers in vaccines that are then injected into our children! We all have subtle energy fields, which I will describe in depth a little later, and our energy fields respond to things like mercury. Subtle energy is conducted more easily and quickly than the electrical energy that is found in our nervous systems. Our subtle energy systems also react to the electromagnetic energy that is thrown from power lines and other environmental factors, as well as electronics, computers, and even electromagnetic emissions from the planet Earth.

Subtle Energy Fields and Harmonics

As the conductive filler substances in the vaccines enter the body, even in tiny doses, our subtle energy systems respond, and when they do, a couple of things might happen. First of all, the body's energy system may become disharmonic in an effort to normalize in response to the introduction of the substance. Secondly, because our consciousness is actually pure energy, when the conductive materials are injected in their little bodies, children's subtle fields of energy expand and there is not enough room for the consciousness to completely seat in the body or the head. Because of that, literally *part of the conscious awareness of that child is no longer present in the body but living at varying degrees outside the body.* The distance and effect depends upon the harmonics of that individual in the first place, which is why the autism spectrum of symptoms and effects is so wide.

Secondary to the energy field responding to the physical pollution brought on by the vaccine fillers comes a response from the autoimmune system. Since, as we will learn later, the digestive tract is the lowest frequency part of our energy system, our autoimmune system literally attacks the digestive system in error because the harmonics become abnormal, thus causing atypical reactions to foods, drugs, environment, and other stimuli. Digestive symptoms are a common experience in autistic people, especially children.

Autism continues to be considered a mystery and a blanket diagnosis for a spectrum of early childhood dysfunction. From an alternative point of view, this spectrum of dysfunction is caused by disharmonies in frequencies of the body, and these disharmonies are caused by the introduction of conductive materials to the internal system, either directly or environmentally.

I have come to realize that our bodies learn from their experiences. Our DNA learns how to instruct us in the future based upon its current and past experiences. Our energy constantly shifts and changes in response to both internal and external stimuli. Our life experiences are literally responses to the condition of our energy fields and our experiences that change those fields.

Further examples of effects to the subtle energy field contributing to illness or states of being are so-called diseases such as schizophrenia and other mental disorders, multiple sclerosis (MS), cancer, and virtually every disease presently known. Each has a cause and an effect based upon the subtle energy system. Sometimes these problems occur because the system is out of harmony with what would be its norm. Other times these problems happen because parts of the harmonics are overstimulated or missing.

For instance, in the case of schizophrenia, the "filters" that weed out altered or other-dimensional reality information from our human experience are not working correctly or, in severe cases, are missing altogether. Certain medications help with this but do not treat the original cause. In this case, the body is responding to the missing "filters" by producing errors in brain chemical production.

A greatly contributing factor to multiple sclerosis is overstimulation of the subtle energy field that then translates to the electrical (nerve) system and creates dysfunction. When MS symptoms occur acutely, it is because the system has begun looping energetically in specific areas, and as a result, the entire subtle energy system becomes red and inflamed. Then, following the inflammation of the subtle energy, physical symptoms and an errant electrical system occur.

Cancer is a responsive disease, which basically results from mutations of cells due to a variety of reasons or to stimuli within the body. These mutated cells become dense and misunderstood by normal body systems, so they become dangerous to the body as a whole. In other words, cancer functions as an outsider to the generally attuned energy system. The mutated areas develop individual sets of harmonics that live within yet are foreign to the body. The autoimmune system tries to fight it but does not generally succeed because it does not recognize the harmonics within the cancerous area.

Harmonics apply to most every illness or affliction of the body. One of the most interesting things that I learned when reading bodies is that even though an organ, such as an appendix, a gallbladder, or a uterus, may have been removed, the original energy field of that organ remains. The energy field is so strong that it is often difficult to tell whether or not the organ has been removed. If the organ had been dysfunctional to any degree, the energy of the dysfunction remains in the body, and the person may continue to experience symptoms even after the organ's removal via surgery.

A Complete Picture: Conventional and Complementary Medicine

So why consider allopathic medicine if we know such great alternatives exist? One point that I want to make perfectly clear before proceeding any further in this book is that to put aside allopathic medicine completely is as big a mistake as it is to deny that alternative methods don't exist or don't work. There are many aspects to our being. Besides our emotional, mental and spiritual bodies, we have a physical body that must at times be treated in a manner to which it will respond: physically. Over the years I have met people who are of the metaphysical belief that they have the power to heal themselves and that doctors will only contribute to worsening their situations.

Absolutely, alternative healing works. At least what I have experienced and seen does, and I am sure that other modalities work just as well. Absolutely and without a doubt, we can heal ourselves; however, self healing to the degree that disease goes away and the body is perfectly and forever healed takes a level of self-mastery that few achieve.

We can believe with all of our hearts and souls that we will be well and maybe we will. I know it can be so. I am living proof. But I also have seen people become extremely ill, and even die, from what began as a minor problem, because they became infected, or the problem grew in form or its effects grew worse, when a simple visit to their doctor in the beginning could have cleared up the problem quickly. Honestly, I have seen people die because they didn't want to go to a physician because they thought they could handle the problem themselves. Unfortunately, in those cases, the problem went way beyond any kind of help and then it was too late.

As long as we are human beings, we live in a biological physicality that is subject to invasion and infestation by viruses, bacteria, parasites, and other pesky problems. Sometimes people don't go to the doctor because they are afraid of what they might find out. At other times, money issues or lack of insurance keep them from seeking medical help. No matter the excuse, the truth is that everyone deserves care. Sometimes a visit to our family doc can take care of those things quickly. Other times our local alternative healer can help. Sometimes we are sicker than we realize, but we are afraid to face a real diagnosis. The dread of not knowing or our denial that it exists at all can be much worse than the reality of having the problem treated. In fact, not facing fear of the unknown can actually draw to us exactly what we feared.

Allopathic and alternative medicines can work together in a complementary manner in which the patient receives a holistic form of care from all directions. Sometimes, depending upon circumstances, one kind of treatment may outweigh the other. Just as we need to be open to and accepting of alternative health care, we also need to be open to medical treatment. To me, each situation dictates its needs. I completely advocate alternative healing whenever possible. It can be even more effective than allopathic medicine because it can treat aspects of our being that allopathic medicine never even considers.

Sometimes our illnesses become our identity, and when that happens the battle to cure them can become unwinnable. What we believe becomes reality. Treating the client holistically, no matter what path of treatment is chosen, is the highest and best route in every case. Treating just the symptoms doesn't alleviate the cause. Treating the obvious physical cause does not treat the more subtle aspects of any illness.

The bottom line is if something isn't working for you, do what does work; know when to make those choices and don't hesitate to make them. If you choose alternative care, believe in it, find someone who is knowledgeable and responsible, and don't hop from one healer to another. With energy work in particular, every time someone else accesses your energy field, whatever the previous healer did becomes interrupted and may no longer be in place. Even if their modalities are different, they are still working within the energy field. It is easy to have the body harmonics knocked so far out of whack that we really do get worse. Don't look for Band-Aids or quick fixes because they don't work. Instead, invest in yourself. *Know* that you are well. *Believe* that you are well. No one can fix you if you aren't willing to accept the fixing. Know that you are healing and healed.

If you desire allopathic medicine, so be it, but get more than one opinion, and don't allow yourself to be frightened into a radical decision. Become invested in yourself and the outcome. Don't give your healing power to anyone. It begins with you.

Alternative choices are up to you, the client, the patient, and no one else. No matter what you choose, no judgment should be rendered. Always be open to new and different ideas and forms of treatment even if they seem strange or are unknown to you. Sometimes an alternative choice can change your life. Miracles happen every day; sometimes they just need a little help.

CHAPTER TWO

What Does It Take to Be a Good Healer?

In all good conscience, I couldn't write a book about healing of any kind without addressing what it means to be a good healer. Healing modalities are often approached with a checklist of skills and opinions that have been generated about the client either in advance of the session or by what is learned in the process of the session. A healer may have passed tests, taken classes, or have certain perceptions, but who is the healer as a person? True healing requires holistic treatment of the body, mind, spirit, and soul. To me, being a good healer begins with an open mind and heart and a willingness to stretch beyond any preconceptions to *really see and hear* the client.

Too many times I have encountered alternative healers who feel that whatever results the client receives are solely the doing of the healer. Worse, many healers are attached to the outcome and blame themselves if the healing that was intended doesn't take place. Let's talk about what it takes to be a truly good healer.

We Must Deal with Our Own Issues before Ever Touching Another Soul

First of all, when we use whatever healing modality we have learned or know, it is vital to remain in humility. We are conduits for grace. When we step into the mode of Etheric healing, we intentionally join the One to work from within creation rather than at it. Creation is filled with infinite possibilities that are available to us to bring forward for the specific assistance of our clients. When we can remain as open vessels for the energies of creation to flow through us, as you will learn how to do later in this book, there is absolutely no question that those energies will go wherever they are needed. Further, the energies that come through us will adapt based upon our client's needs. To confuse pure grace with human nature can lead to difficult times for any healer. Questioning what we are doing in the moments of healing is like calling in God and then questioning his judgment.

When we are doing healing work, it is vital that we stay clear, having dealt with our own issues so that we don't confuse them with the issues of others. I have met a lot of healers who like to use their session time talking all about their own problems and experiences and commiserating with their clients. They identify with every complaint the client has. This is a great big no-no. Our clients don't come to hear our problems and issues. They come because they need something that they aren't getting in their lives. We have set ourselves to help them find what they need and to help them overcome their challenges. We need to remember that.

To me, one of the greatest traits a good healer can have it to listen deeply to what the client is really saying. Often it is between the words where the truth lies. In order to be a good listener, we must be comfortable letting our defenses down and really be open to our clients. When we are defensive in any way, we will never hear anything our clients say that is relevant to our own issues. Instead, we become tense and tight, and our energy does not flow well. Our minds get in the way and we can't hear our clients' deeper truths. Allowing our intuition to take over sets the stage for greater honesty and deeper work.

What we must remember is that energy always exchanges. Let me repeat that: energy always exchanges. When we encounter anyone anywhere and interact with them, no matter how briefly, some of our energy enters the other person's field and some of their energy enters ours. After every encounter we have, we never, ever, walk away exactly the same as we arrived. By encountering and interacting in no matter how limited a way with another, we are re-harmonized. No matter how we feel, what we experience, how we perceive our interactions with others, no matter how brief, we are affected, as are they. It is important to remember that if our issues are getting the best of us and we are not feeling balanced, we should never touch anyone else in the name of healing. The kind of work we will be learning later in this book is so clean, so pure, that it can carry any message into the energy field and, therefore, into the body of our client.

Good Communication Is Vital

It is true that communication is a two-way street, but this is more true than we ever considered. When we communicate with others, we do so, not only with our words, but also with our bodies and our energy systems. With every word we say, energy follows. Energy is the word. It is the meaning of the word. Energy is in how the word is heard and how it is applied on the receiving end. As we communicate, subtle energy moves toward the other person and literally enters their energy field. Conversely, when we listen to another, it is not just their words that we receive. We receive their intentions, their motivations, the energy of their communication, and, if we are listening, perhaps even their actual message. We do this with our ears and our cognitive senses and also with our energy fields. Our energy fields then rearrange and harmonize based upon the message we receive.

A good listener does not distract herself with random thoughts or self-defensiveness but, rather, focuses directly on the messenger, diligently listening to hear the true message that usually comes between the lines of communication.

Honesty

As part of our subconscious defense system, we learn early on to avoid telling ourselves the truth that we don't want to hear. As we move through our lives, not telling ourselves the truth may have evolved into not telling others the truth as well. We learn to smooth things over or avoid them completely. Sometimes we just don't talk about what we are really feeling.

To be a good healer we must come clean with ourselves. If we can't allow ourselves to recognize our own stuff, we aren't going to clearly hear someone else's. When clients come for healing, they are seeking something. It becomes our job as a healer to know what our clients really want. If we are unclear with ourselves, we aren't clear with our clients either. Healing doesn't just fix physical issues; it changes lives.

A good thing to remember about honesty and telling the truth is that the message is always dependent upon the messenger. If we are sincere and honest, calm and caring, about how we share information with our clients, what we share will be heard more fully and even utilized long after our clients have left the building.

A good rule of thumb is not to barrage the client with information, but instead to tell them what is pertinent, what matters. Often when our intuitive nature opens with a client, we may receive tons of information. We must be willing and responsible enough to be discerning about how and what we communicate.

An extreme example of this is when we witness something in a person's Etheric field that indicates that they will die soon. Sometimes fixing a physical problem isn't our job, but helping that person through the challenge is. What isn't our job *ever* is to tell a client what their experience is or *should* be.

A healer wields a lot of power in this department. I can't tell you how many times I have met people whose entire lives are falling apart because they are trying to be something that someone else told them they were. People take to heart what we tell them as if our words have some magic that makes things true. We must be very careful not to lead someone into an experience that might not have otherwise been theirs.

Sometimes the Whole Truth Is Too Much

Once in a while, it is hard to know how much to say and how much not to say. If I sense that a person has a tumor or some vital illness and it doesn't appear that what we are doing is changing the problem, I lovingly tell them—not every single one of my impressions—but that I am sensing something that perhaps they may want to follow up on with their medical doctor. Never, *ever*, would I tell a person they only had so long to live. I don't feel that it is my place to take away their hope. There are times when a situation looks dreary, but then hope and belief in a different outcome saves lives. I would also not tell a client that their disease was terminal . . . unless they directly asked me. My policy is to be directly but lovingly honest when asked, even when the answers are hard to give. In giving those answers, though, I always leave room for the miracles I know are possible!

For instance, sometimes fixing someone just isn't our job. We might realize that a person is having an experience that isn't ours to interfere with. Every once in a while that happens. In those situations, there is usually a much greater picture than we can know, or if we do know, we realize that it is much bigger than we are.

For instance, I knew of a boy who, as a result of the devastating damage and ensuing filth and spread of disease in stagnant waters after Hurricane Katrina, fell desperately ill. He was from a small community where everyone knew everyone. He and his dad and others had gone wading into the floodwaters in order to check what was left of their home and to search for survivors. Days later the boy became very, very sick. No one could seem to figure out what was wrong with him, and as his fever rose, his life force withered.

Everyone involved wondered why him, how could that be? And to such a nice family. The focus became his illness, what it was, how to stop it, how to cure the boy. But this time was one of those where the whole picture is much greater.

As first the boy, then the family, then immediate friends, then others, and finally, the community were affected by the illness and later passing of this brave young soul, their lives changed forever in their relations to each other and how they learned to see the world through the eyes of the dying boy. His messages will travel far and wide, indelibly remaining in the hearts of not only those he touched but everyone around him. His death changed an entire community.

Our job may be to listen to our clients, coach them though their tough situation, assist in relieving symptoms, or just tell them the truth no one else will but only ever in response to their asking. Sometimes fixing people just isn't ours to do.

Telling someone that they will die in the next three weeks (and, yes, the information can get very specific) is not okay. Doing so would just about guarantee that three weeks to the day later, that person will leave the planet. Instead, perhaps the thing to honestly say is that they may want get their affairs in order, say what they need to say, or if possible, do what they have left undone.

Telling a person he is terminally ill isn't always ours to do either. That takes away all hope and limits the possibility of any other outcome for them. The power of the mind and of belief is one of the greatest aspects of healing in creation. We need to leave open the possibility that healing may occur. Sometimes believing is enough.

What if, in that situation, there had been other possibilities; what if the course of that person's life could have gone differently; what if a spontaneous cure or a change in the course of the disease were possible? If we had told that person definitely and without a doubt that a certain reality would happen, our message would have become the only possibility the client could see.

If a person who is fighting for his life asks me how long or when, I tell him (even if I know) that that answer isn't mine to give, that each and every moment is a gift, and to live it fully. If someone wants confirmation that they are terminally ill, I might answer a direct yes, or, depending upon the client, I might answer that that is how things look at this time but that miracles happen every day and we don't need to set the illness in the concrete of our beliefs. Whenever possible, always leave room for a different outcome. It is in those seemingly slim chances that miracles seem to appear out of nowhere.

The greatest thing to remember is that the truth is *our* interpretation, always. We must realize that the truth may often have many facets. How we tell that truth and how it is heard is largely up to us.

Integrity and Compassion

A good healer must absolutely have the highest values of integrity, first to self, then to the client. The process of healing may at times bring up lot of drama and trauma. We aren't there to play into that, only to address what needs to be addressed, and to be unconditionally compassionate with our clients. If we haven't learned to be compassionate with ourselves, we surely can't be compassionate with our clients. To me, compassion is a huge part of integrity.

Our healing space is sacred. What happens there stays there. We have no right to share the intimate things we learn about our clients with anyone else. We have no right to have an opinion about how they are handling things, only to help our client learn to do things differently. As we will learn later, the body and its energy fields tell a complete story about the person with whom we work. That is their story.

We must learn to be comfortable enough to answer the client's questions truthfully; otherwise, we aren't giving them what they came for. How we answer those questions must be truthful yet leave the outcome to whatever possibilities may be available.

Boundaries Are Important and So Is Our Value

When we learn to Touch the Light, to work within creation to bring change into the lives of others, it is vital that we learn to take care of ourselves in the process. When I first learned how to do this work, word got around fast that miracles were happening. All of a sudden everyone seemed to have an emergency that they believed only I could fix. Soon my phone was ringing 24/7. People were knocking at my door at all hours; if I didn't answer right away, some even looked into my windows. At first, I didn't know how to say no, or gee, they didn't really have an emergency and whatever it was could wait until a time that was convenient for me. Needless to say, I got tired. I began to wonder where my life had gone because suddenly it was about everyone else. Something had to change. Not only was I doing a disservice to myself, but also to my clients.

I learned to make appointments around my schedule. I also learned what true emergencies were and if possible made myself available for them. I learned that if I didn't eat and sleep I wasn't much good for anyone else. I also learned the very valuable lesson that I had value and if I was going to be able to continue with the healing, I had to have some sort of exchange in order to sustain my life. I learned that it was okay to charge for my time. Many of those who were just looking for attention quickly fell away, and those in real need came. As an aside, I realized that people really do get what they pay for, and those who invested in themselves by paying me for my time were much more diligent in their recovery.

There is a great urban legend that to do spiritual work means to be barefoot and poor. That isn't spiritual; that is insane. We deserve to be compensated fairly for our time. Then we have the resources to work unhindered by stressful money issues. In all of that realization, though, I never turned away anyone who honestly could not pay for my time. I found great reward, time and time again, by quietly helping those in real need. Payment in those cases was far greater than any dollar could have ever been, and it still is.

Leave Your Ego at the Door

Once we have learned to Touch the Light, many things happen. Miracles happen. People's lives change because this kind of healing work touches every level of a person's being in body, mind, and spirit, even beyond. We must remember that these changes are not from us; they are of us. We are not giving ourselves away when we perform healing; we are conduits for energy in the form of what I must call grace. That energy knows what to do, where to do it, and every intricate detail that is involved in the healing process. It is fueled by our intentions. We are sharing ourselves in this giving way, but only sharing. Not being, not doing. What comes out of a healing session is really up to the person receiving the work. Does she believe in it? Is she willing to accept the changes that can come to her? Is he really asking for what he needs or just what he thinks he wants? We, the healers, can only make available to the client what comes through us at their request. It is the job of the recipient to accept and apply the work. For a healer to have any ego at all about Touching the Light is to be completely out of truth.

Take Time to Regenerate

Anytime we deal with others on any level, we give part of ourselves. Each and every one of us must learn to receive as easily as we give. To receive is an admission of value. To receive keeps the cycle of energy flowing. We must be willing and open to allowing ourselves to regenerate our own energy and comfort in order to remain as strong and effective healers.

Human vs. Spirit

One of the most difficult issues that many effective healers has is becoming confused between their divinity and their humanity. Often we tend to see our humanity as something outside of or separate from ourselves. What we don't realize is that we are divine creatures who are created from all things and all things are created of us. We are intricately woven into the fabric of reality and have the innate ability to create from the infinite possibilities that are available to us by virtue of our connection.

In confusing divinity and humanity, I have literally seen many budding healers and intuitives become victims of their own giftedness. When we begin to see real-time events occur that we envisioned ahead of time, or when we literally see lives change as a result of our touch, these are powerful reminders that something is happening that is far greater than we can comprehend. These things are not separate at all. They are part of who we are. When we become more open to our gifts, our gifts become more open. As they do, our perceptions become wider and wider and far different from what was in our limited past. Because of this, it is easy to become entangled in religious or social beliefs that conflict with the paranormal. The truth is that we have discovered, and some day science will agree, that all normal is paranormal and that reality is nothing more than the perception of our experience.

To embrace our gifts is to embrace our true being. Just because we have these gifts doesn't set us apart; quite the opposite. We rejoin the One from the inside out. In a way, we marry our divinity to our humanity, becoming attuned to the possibilities of what it means to be unlimited.

Just because we use our inherent talents does not make us responsible for the entire world. Nor does it mean we have to give ourselves away until we drop. Using our gifts simply means being who we are.

Know Your Local Legalities

Along with knowing the local legalities, we must always remember that we are not medical doctors and should not act as such. Advising people about their prescriptions, doctor's orders, and other medically prescribed therapies is not generally within our realm of expertise. Doing so is usually breaking the law and can inadvertently harm our clients.

Instead, when we receive information about a client that is applicable or advisable related to a medical condition, I highly suggest that we advise him to check with his medical doc before changing or discontinuing prescriptions. If our advice is in the area of a medical concern, most of us are not medical doctors, and it is best to be honest, make suggestions, make sure that our clients know they have a choice in all of their medical experiences, but leave the final decisions up to our clients. We can certainly share our impressions, our thoughts, and interpretations of the same matters, but giving actual medical advice is against the law unless we are licensed physicians.

Every state, country, and local venue has laws to protect the public. Some of these laws may apply particularly to hands on healing. Some laws require licensure while others are more lenient and still others forbid it altogether. Make certain that you are familiar with the laws in your area and that you adhere to their requirements.

Sometimes laws can be circumvented by having a designation as clergy or by ordination as a minister. Far more protection may come under these designations than an individual hanging a shingle out. This point is vitally important so that at some point healers do not find themselves in precarious legal situations.

It is also good to get to know other healers and medical personnel in your area so that you can develop a referral network. The best advertising is word of mouth and that goes both ways. If the medical people in your area see that your work is not only responsible, but also getting good results, they are less likely to see you as a quack. Over time, because of my respect for the work of others and their opinions, I not only gleaned infinitely valuable information, I also began to receive active referrals from medical doctors of varying specialties, psychologists, psychiatrists, massage therapists, chiropractors, and others. Later, many of them asked me to assist them and their families with problems they were otherwise unable to resolve. Mutuality is a terrific tool to create a thriving practice in your area. Hanging out a laundry list of achieved designations doesn't prove anything either. We must be who we say we are as well as walk our talk and be an example of the possibilities we know are real.

CHAPTER THREE

Becoming Well:
Band-Aids and Miracles

Healing has always been a great mystery, especially when a cure works for one person but perhaps not for another. Part of the success or failure of any healing modality is how the recipient perceives and accepts the healing.

Let's face it. Some of us believe unconditionally in being well, whole, and happy while others seem to be stuck in their misery. Some people use illness and pain as a way to get attention, while others see their illness as their identity. When these types of things are happening, it becomes difficult to change the situation because the pain or illness has literally become part of the person's belief system. We will learn more about the hows and whys of this later, but for now, think of it like this: When we become injured or ill, the first thing that happens is that we literally clamp down on the injury or illness. We hold our breath. We become tense. The reality of the moments sinks in, and then we become emotional. We embrace the symptoms as something we can't help, and then we see the thing as controlling our lives—so it does. One minute we thought everything was fine, and the next minute we see ourselves as imperfect, sick, or injured.

Why Some People Heal and Others Don't

How we approach and experience our illnesses and injuries has everything to do with the outcome. Early on I learned a very little thing that proved to be huge in my comprehension of healing. I realized that if I could treat an injury immediately after its occurrence, that injury would heal in record time; often, it would be as if it had never happened in the first place. As the emotions became involved, the injury became more ingrained and therefore a much more difficult experience to heal. I came to realize how much our emotions are involved in our experiences of health and healing. When we tense and become afraid of what is happening to us, we literally condense the energy surrounding the situation. As the energy becomes denser, the possibilities of quick and full healing become less and less. The experience becomes our identity and, therefore, the reality that continues to be experienced.

A simple example of this theory came one day in the form of a series of hornet stings that happened to a little boy at my friend's home. He came in screaming, and it was quickly obvious that he had been stung multiple times all over his legs. Welts were rising, and his legs were already an angry red.

He was sitting on the floor screaming and crying in a lot of pain. He was feeling helpless, as children often do when they are injured. I quietly got down behind him and calmly talked to him. I told him that he didn't need to keep those mean old stings and then I don't know what possessed me, but I asked him to give the stings to me and assured him that they wouldn't hurt me. His first reaction was to fight with me, to pull away in his fear. His second response was priceless.

The crying stuttered to a stop and he looked at me through his tears, his eyebrows raised as if to ask, "Are you for real?" I returned his gaze, and we shared a wordless moment of knowing together. He began to relax, and I began to pull the energy of the stings out of his small legs. I asked the little guy to help me by letting go of the stings, and within minutes the stings were gone and he had forgotten all about his earlier misadventure with the hornets. He didn't have a mark on him where before his legs had already turned an angry red and were swollen. Left untreated, the stings would have grown into painful itchy areas that would have lasted for days if not longer, damaging the tissue around the area of the stings. This experience fascinated me and opened up a plethora of possibilities to consider in regard to how and why people get well.

Time and again, I witnessed similar situations where an injury occurred and then disappeared with immediate energy work. Instead of putting energy in, I pulled it out. The results were burns with no blisters, bumps and scrapes with no bruises or bleeding, and, later, tumors that began to grow then disappeared, and many other events just as amazing in their results in both simple and complex situations.

There it was, time and again, the body responding beautifully to healing, and I had to seriously consider what was being shown to me. I began to explore how fear and emotion dictated the outcome of physical circumstances. That led me to learn how the energy field, and then the physical body, responds to fear and emotion, which led me to begin to understand why some people are able to become well easily while others seem to struggle and some never get well at all. It all factors down to how we experience the initial information or event. Fear and emotion are immense factors in times of injury and illness. The more quickly fear and other emotions enter the picture, the more difficult it can be to change the situation as a healer, but most of the time it is still possible.

Our reaction to our circumstances nearly always dictates the experience and its outcome. Yes, we have that much power in our own process.

When Illness or Injury Can't Be Fixed—Sometimes the Reasons Are Greater Than Us and Dying Is Okay

Sometimes there are circumstances that we aren't meant to change or heal. Sometimes it is time for a soul to move on in its journey. Life is like that. We have, throughout our lives, windows of opportunity through which we can transition right on out of our earthly lives. Dying is part of living, and it is inevitable when we are in human form. Dying is nothing to fear and everything to celebrate. After all, a life has been lived; we have experienced that soul in different capacities as family, lovers, friends, and other relationships. Each relationship has memories that are ours forever.

Some cultures, like the Toltec's in Mexico and others in Central and South America, teach that death is looking over our shoulder all the time. The question is, are we ready? That is a little scary at first, but when we consider the lesson in that knowledge, we immediately feel our resistance and our self-deceptions regarding the subject of dying. What we can learn from knowing that death could take us at any time is to live fully every moment as if it is the only one we have. To not save things for special occasions but instead to make everything a special occasion. Too many times people lose opportunities that were right there in front of them because they thought it would be better to wait for later. There is only ever this now. What was has been, and what hasn't yet been is either imagination or speculation. Go for it!

Sometimes the illness itself is not as much about the person who experiences it as it is about those who are affected around that person. Like the example I gave earlier about the little boy who died from a disease he caught after Hurricane Katrina, sometimes the effects of the situation change others so profoundly that they will never see their lives the same again. It happens.

The courage and dignity that some people exhibit when they know they are about to leave the planet can be profound. So can the fear. So can the reasons themselves. It is beyond difficult to go through the ravages of some injuries and diseases. What sharing these events does to the families, friends, and others leaves an indelible mark on everyone involved. When their perceptions are changed, they live and treat others differently. Those actions may ripple outward from one person to the next until there is no longer a way to track just how much the illness or death of a single person can touch others. I have come to know that these types of situations may be Karmic in nature. Maybe, just maybe, the one person who affected so many was playing a part in a much grander scheme of things.

Band-Aids—Healing to Get Attention

Early on in my healing practice I realized that some people seek attention with their illnesses. As I began to meet and treat more and more people, some of them wanted to return time and time again. I realized that they saw the sickness, whatever it was, as their way to get attention. I call this "comfortable discomfort." There are always reasons we see ourselves as imperfect or damaged, and I found that in those situations it wasn't really about the illness; it was more often about emotional pain that wasn't being addressed.

I found myself in the role of counselor as well as healer. In these instances I found that simple direct conversations helped these clients to completely change their outlooks. I believe it is better to empower clients rather than enable them to need. Always, always, I give people possibilities whenever and however I can find them.

There are also those who just want to stay unhappy and are unwilling to do what it takes to change their circumstances. Some would return every day or every week if I let them. This kind of work can be instantaneous and permanent, so too many repeat sessions indicate an ongoing problem or a client's unwill-ingness to participate in the changes that would bring her to fuller healing. I decided that if, after three sessions, no improvement was noted I would refer a client to someone more suited to their immediate needs. In some cases I would simply have an honest conversation about my perception of the situation, shar-ing alternative perspectives and suggestions that they could use to turn their life around. Of course, I always told them that when they were ready to do their part, I would be there to help them make the changes they desired. Just having that conversation was often the beginning of a great turnaround for them. If they still didn't listen or improve I simply stopped seeing them.

To Experience a Miracle, We Must Have Passion

I have already mentioned several occasions when amazing healings occurred. In looking back at some of those moments I realize that the person receiving the healing was fully present and had a complete unadulterated desire to be well or healed. I also realized that my level of passion was at indescribable heights. As a healer, I couldn't have been more connected with my clients and they with the process. Every moment of those experiences was unconditional in every way. Even with new clients I had never met before, life changed immediately and dra-matically because we were so in sync and intentional about the outcome of the session. They believed, desired, wanted, and needed to heal. I believed, desired, and knew that they could.

Passion is the driving force of all intention. When we work from our heart spaces, we are utilizing the forces of creation in such a pure way that the intention is cleanly communicated and received. Any kind of healing process that comes from a purely mental state cannot be fully successful because the emotion isn't present.

CHAPTER FOUR

Our Seventh Sense:
God Consciousness and How It Works

Our thinking self and our conscious self work hand-in-hand most of the time, but are not at all the same thing. Our brain works basically as a very low voltage electrical system that is wired by nerve cells (neurons) and their synapses (the spaces between them). When our brain is stimulated, messages quickly fire along the nerve paths, and we react accordingly. Some of the activities of our nervous system are voluntary, while others are not. Our mental selves are electrical in both action and reaction. Without the working webs of nerves in our bodies, we would not be functional at all on a physical level; we would not even be alive.

At the same time our nerves are working to support us, electromagnetic fields are created. Electromagnetic energy is our life force, also known as *chi*. This force enters through our crown, at the very tops of our heads, and flows down through our pranic tube, which is a large pathway right down through the center of our bodies. This invisible force animates our bodies and moves through us continually via our meridian systems. Our meridian systems are invisible highways that weave through our bodies. Along our meridian lines are power points that are relative to different areas of our body and its health. Some of these power points are related to our internal organs, while others are related to different aspects of our health and physical experience. Throughout our entire bodies, as well as around our bodies, fields of energy are emitted all of the time. When we are happy, excited, feeling good, or generally experiencing life in a positive way, our energy fields are large, even expansive. When we are sick, tired, or in a negative frame of mind, our energy fields become much smaller and less vital.

Electromagnetic energy is not simply an invisible force, though. It is a conscious living thing, filled with information that it transmits and receives both from us and to us. That information is part of our consciousness.

Consciousness is not bound by any walls or defined areas. It is *super luminal*, or faster than the speed of light. It is not bound by direction but can be directed. It is not subject to time and space but can travel through and beyond it, and it is not just some nebulous thing in our heads; it is everywhere in our bodies.

Consciousness is awake and aware 24/7, and it experiences not only what is happening in our bodies and our minds, but also in all of creation. Consciousness never forgets anything because all information that passes through our consciousness is retained in a form that is very different from our neuron-oriented electrical brains.

Gamma Consciousness and Our Seventh Sense

Our brains perform different kinds of activity. This activity is measured in waves, such as alpha (when we are relaxed), beta (active awareness), delta (when we are sleeping) and theta (when we meditate and get "out there"). These are the most common types of brain waves, but there is one other type that is not as well understood. It is called the gamma wave.

Gamma brain waves can be found in virtually all areas of the brain. In fact, they serve to unify all of our senses so that we can see, hear, smell, feel,

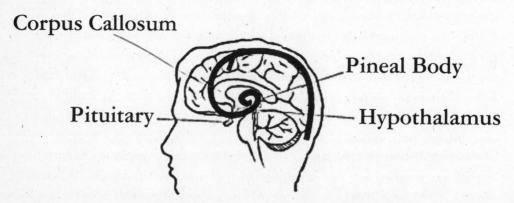

The spiral of consciousness incorporates every major part of our brain.

and taste all at once. Gamma waves are the fastest known type of brain waves. They are so subtle that they are barely discernible on an electroencephalogram (EEG), or brain wave test. Gamma waves are thought to be used during our most purely cognitive brain state. They also assist in expansion of reality perception, increased I.Q, improved states of consciousness, more physical energy, and positive thinking, as well as other benefits.

I discovered during the expansion of my awareness that during different levels of consciousness there are actually three levels of gamma wave states. I call these initiation, communion, and ascension. These levels of consciousness occur when certain aspects of our brain wave activity unify to create increasingly higher levels of awareness. When we enter into any level of gamma wave activity, we are stimulated along a predictable spiral in our brains. That spiral encompasses our pineal gland, pituitary gland, corpus callosum (the dividing point in the center of our brains), and our hypothalamus, up across the crown of our heads and around to the back of our skull between the occipital bones. The first level of Gammas Consciousness, Initiation, is at the widest part of the spiral at the back of the head. At the point that the arc of the spiral crosses the crown, the Communion phase of consciousness is reached. With each level of Gamma Consciousness, we come closer to having full unification of energy in our brain. Full unification of the brain's energy field occurs when the center point of the spiral is activated during extremely high awareness. At that point the third level of Gamma Consciousness is reached, and we arrive at the highest aspect of consciousness, which is the ascension point.

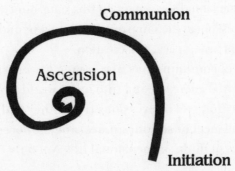

The three levels of Gamma Consciousness.

Initiation

The first level of Gamma Consciousness is what I call initiation. It is at this level of awareness that we begin to realize that there are realities beyond our considered norm. This state of consciousness is where we most use our sixth sense. Our sixth sense is our intuitive nature. It is how we know something is going to happen before it does, how we know who is on the phone just before it rings, how we know things about people we haven't been told, and many other instances when our consciousness is used in paranormal circumstances.

At the initiation level, we might begin to have flashes of visions of past, present, or future events. Our intuition is awakened, and with it we may begin to see, hear, or feel snippets of other realities. This stage of awareness is that at which we think we see something or someone out the corner of our eye that isn't really there, at least not in our "regular" world.

Communion

The communion level of Gamma Consciousness occurs when the gamma wave energy expands through the crown of our head and connects with the incoming energies that are entering our pranic tube. Gamma consciousness is not only the combining of our senses, but the unification of our brain waves so that for the time we are in that state, we are literally accessing all of the parts of our brain, including those we rarely use. The energy that is incoming through our crown carries information about everything that ever is, was, or will be. It is here, at the communion stage of consciousness, that our Seventh Sense becomes activated. Our Seventh Sense is our inter-dimensional awareness. In this state, our consciousness remains connected to our bodies, but at the same time freely roams and communicates across all boundaries of time, space, and creation.

Being in the state of communion is like having your cosmic antennae extended past the third dimension and into other worlds, receiving direct downloads of information and impressions from other realities. In the communion stage, we may meet or see our guides, angels, deceased people in spirit form, and other forms of multi-dimensional life. Not only that, we can communicate with them.

When the Masters came to me and we interacted so closely, I was in the communion state. It was an easy connection, fluid and ongoing until I chose to do something else (like go to work) each day. It became extremely easy (and still is) to connect to otherworldly realities.

In addition to communicating and interacting multi-dimensionally, our Seventh Sense also allows for our consciousness to travel unhindered into other levels of reality. When using our Seventh Sense, we are also able to travel through star gate systems in the same way that our ancient intergalactic ancestors did. Traveling the star gate systems isn't necessarily only about jumping from star system to star system. The network of connections that is available throughout the multiverse includes corridors, dimensional portals, and wormholes, all of which can be accessed by our consciousness while using our Seventh Sense. Making and maintaining this connection is kind of like being online all the time.

As healers, using our Seventh Sense can create the fullest, most effective, alternative healing possible.

Ascension

Ascension consciousness is the third level of Gamma Consciousness. It occurs when our brain waves are unified, our thinking brain is disengaged, and the entire electromagnetic system inside and around our bodies has unified all at the same time. This only happens when we have achieved a certain level of awareness that we not only sustain, but also literally become a part of.

When we achieve this level of consciousness, our DNA strands begin to emit stronger and stronger electromagnetic fields of energy until there comes a moment when every single strand of DNA in our bodies is unified energetically.

As this occurs, our consciousness links, not only with the communion field of Gamma Consciousness energy, but also with the electromagnetic energy that is emitted within our bodies. At that point we achieve the embodiment of a true trinity. This trinity consists of us as an individual, our connection with Creation, and the combination of ourselves with creation. It is at this point of consciousness that we have the ability to turn to white light and disappear, taking our bodies right along with us.

Exercise One: Movement to Spirit

Movement to Spirit is the exercise that came out of my own desperation to learn about and process the huge amounts of energy that were flowing through my body early in my awakening process. I laughingly called it my personal brand of tai chi. I have taught this exercise to every one of my classes often with profound results. If done correctly (hard not to) and with no expectations at all, this exercise can help you go from earthbound to multi-dimensional in no time at all.

Step One: Find some music that moves your heart. You know, the kind that makes your heart feel expanded and overall emotional. It is best not to use hemi-sync (brain balancing) music or music that has words when you first begin. Brain wave music will actually keep you from experiencing the leap to gamma state. Words carry energy of their own and make the music more complex.

Music becomes an actual part of us while we are listening to it. As the music plays, its energy and harmonics fill the environment. That energy signals the particulates within our bodies to temporarily restructure, to move farther apart, allowing the particulates of the music to move through us. In these moments we become changed. The music and we are joined. This is part of why music has such great emotional effect.

When you are ready, begin playing the music.

Step Two: With your eyes closed, hold your hands out in front of you, side by side, (pinky side down) with the palms facing each other and fingers extended (like you see people do when they pray), but without letting your hands touch. Hold your hands close enough together that you can feel the warm energy between them. This energy is your life force and your unique energy in all of creation. The energy that you are holding in your hands is also your consciousness.

Move your hands apart slowly until you can still barely feel the energy but haven't lost awareness of it. It may take some people a little bit longer to find the energy than others. This is not unusual if you have never worked with energy before. Just be patient with yourself. Once you have found the energy you are ready to begin.

Step Three: As the music plays, and with your eyes remaining closed, focus your awareness on the energy that you hold in your hands and nothing else. Begin to move your body and your arms, allowing your hands to move in sync but remaining apart. Sway gently with the rhythm of the music. It is okay to move your feet if you like. Focus on the energy that is between your hands and nothing else. Begin to move your hands farther apart, maintaining your focus.

What happens to the energy when you do this? Does it get smaller? Larger? More intense? Does the feeling change in any other way? Be aware of any changes in the energy as you move. Keep your eyes closed and just let yourself enjoy the experience of the energy changes.

Note: As you continue with this exercise, it is vitally important that you remember to breathe! Your breath is what assists the energy as it flows through your body. It cleanses you, nourishes you, and maintains your internal balance.

You may begin to feel extremely emotional during this exercise. That is fine. It is a natural part of the opening process. As you begin to raise your consciousness, your frequencies, your vibrational rate, also begins to rise. As it does, your body begins to release energies that had been stuck from hidden emotions as well as certain chemicals that trigger the release of emotional stuff that you have tucked away in your body. Breathe through the feelings and let the tears or other emotions flow if they come. Know that you are beginning to access the part of you that remembers your infinite perfection.

Step Four: As the music continues to play, keep your eyes closed, focusing on the energy between your hands just as you did in the previous steps. Now that you have become more comfortable with this process, begin to move more freely, always focusing on the energy between your hands.

Continued

Push the energy outward; let your hands spread further apart as you do. It is okay if you change your hand positions as long as you continue to be aware of the energy with which you are working.

Pull the energy back toward yourself. How does this feel? Is it different than when you push the energy away? As you pull the energy back toward you, try bringing it down over your head. Does this change how you feel? What is your sense? Are you feeling different inside with each movement? Is your awareness to your environment becoming more acute?

Note: As you begin to advance the steps of this exercise, you may experience some pain in certain areas of your body. The areas where you feel pain are telling you that you have an energy blockage there. To remove the blockages, deliberately breathe into the painful area, imagining that your breath is carrying the blockage out of your body as you exhale.

Step Five: *As the music continues to play, keep your eyes closed, focusing on the energy between your hands just as you did in the previous steps. This time as you move, reach as far above your head as you can, bringing the energies down slowly over your head and your body (not touching yourself). Can you feel the subtle changes as you move your hands downward? Now, reach down in front of your feet. Scoop up the energies of the earth and bring them up your legs, your body, and over your head. How do these energies feel different from the ones you brought in from above?*

Step Six: *As the music continues to play, keep your eyes closed, focusing on the energy between your hands just as you did in the previous steps. With a hand just above each hip, pull energy up your sides (still not touching). As you move your hands upward, breathe inward. Do you feel the flow of energy traveling from one chakra center to the next? Can you feel your kundalini, the energy that spirals up around your pranic tube energetic center, awakening? What happens when you deliberately breathe as you move? Does your breath change how the energy feels within or around you?*

Step Seven: *As the music continues to play, keep your eyes closed, focusing on the energy between your hands just as you did in the previous steps. Begin to move freely as you are guided. Always focus only on the energy that is between your hands. Listen to your body and allow it to move with the motion that it desires. Do not feel as if you must remain in one place.*

Move as you will, experiencing the energies as you change position and direction. What effect does direction have on how you perceive the energies? Is there a difference from one direction to another? Allow yourself to naturally move in any way you desire.

The only rules are that you continue to play the music, focus only on the energy that you are working with, and remember to breathe. Remember, this is your experience. Only you will know what movement is most beneficial to you!

This exercise can be done daily for a few minutes or up to an hour as you get stronger. I would not recommend that you do this any more often than that even though it feels awesome. There are changes that are occurring physiologically and energetically within you and around you that will cause you to open in consciousness too quickly if you do this exercise too often. You may deplete minerals that are important to your body such as magnesium and calcium.

You may also become overcharged with energy. This can be very uncomfortable, leaving you feeling as if you are plugged into a cosmic electrical socket somewhere. If this occurs, stop the exercise for a few days and do whatever works best for you to become grounded again. Put your hands in the dirt outside, eat a piece of chocolate, run cold water on your wrists, or even hug a tree. Whatever works for you so that you become grounded and feel completely in your body. It is very easy to become addicted to the sensations that are created by doing this exercise. Remember that the physical sensations are not what this is about. Rather, this is to assist you toward opening to a higher state of conscious awareness.

It is vitally important for you to remember that each time you do this exercise your experiences will be different. If you have an experience one day, don't expect it again the next. Let yourself be open to what comes in each moment. When you do, you are allowing for continued expansion of your awareness.

Also remember that there is no reason to ever, ever, be afraid of what you experience. Remember that this is your experience; you are in control and if you get to a point where your experiences seem too intense, just stop doing the exercise for a few days. Doing it too much can literally open you too quickly!

The Awakening process is an amazing experience. It requires an open heart and mind as well as the willingness to step into new and higher realities. Remember, you get what you ask for! Enjoy the ride!

CHAPTER FIVE

How Consciousness Relates within Creation

If we are to completely understand how consciousness works within the construct of creation, we must first have clarity about how creation is put together. How it is part of us and we are part of it. As I demonstrated in my previous book, *The Secret History of Consciousness*, our ancient predecessors left us brilliantly obvious clues to who we are and what we are capable of. Consciousness and creation

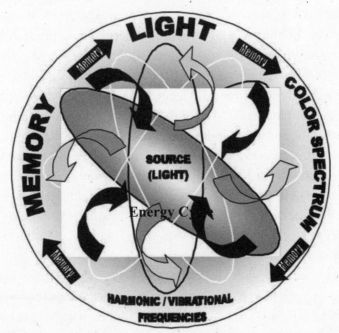

The cycle of energy is never ending. As it is created, it is used up.
As it is used up, it is created.

and their inter-relationships can easily be demonstrated through the use of sacred geometry. Basically, to learn about creation and its relations to our consciousness we have to go back to the very beginning.

The Manifestation of Consciousness in Matter

In the beginning there was no formed mass. All of reality was nothing more than a huge organism of dark material that pulsed and moved in the heart of nothingness. As it did, there were frictional responses that were a lot like static electricity. As the particles rubbed together in the movement of the mass, there were sparks. All at once, the sparks were both an expending and a creation of energy. As more sparks were created, more were used up, and more were created. These were the earliest complete energy cycles. Every spark had a different frequency or set of harmonic frequencies.

The sparks were little tiny forms of light. They had color. They had sound, and no two were identical. As they were used up, the sparks changed frequencies, moving through color spectrums and sound frequencies until they disappeared altogether. As the number of sparks of energy increased within the mass of darkness, they grew in intensity until there came a point in time when the prevalence of light had outgrown the dark matter. The dark matter was pushed outward by the intense energy of the light until at a point in time the balance of the two no longer existed; the light was far greater than the dark matter, and the dark came crashing down upon the light. Some scientists call this the big bang, but it was far more than that. This huge event was the beginning of creation as we know it and the precursor to the formation of matter in every form.

In the moment of this immense cosmic event, the light was dispersed, careening in every direction in a spiral motion. As it did so, in its very being was recorded every moment of its experiences. Each fragment of light recorded similar but wholly different records of its journey.

As the light moved outward, remembering everything from its beginning in the dark matter to every event during its travels, it began to slow down, its initial momentum drained of the original propulsion. As it began to slow, another amazing thing happened. The light began to organize into the first formed realities in creation. It began to first seek other particles like itself that had similar travels and experiences. As the fragments of light began to come together, they continued their spiral motion and began to organize into four-sided pyramids. Each pyramid contained the memory of all of the information it had collected in the form of primitive consciousness, of every fragment that had come together to create it. Because of that, each fragment was literally a formed consciousness. The pyramids became the first organized conscious particles of creation.

Every one of the pyramids contained within it all of the information that each light particle had contributed. The pyramids became the perfect form, as each contained a perfect set of all frequencies of color, light, and sound. No two were identical. Within each pyramid, the memory of the original spiral motion of the fragmented light remained, and a moving spiral of energy formed inside of each pyramid. The spiral spun unendingly, passing information to every fragment of light within its respective pyramid. This action began the manifestation of conscious matter because as the fragments of light within the pyramids received information as they traversed the internal spiral, the light fragments began to respond by changing their order of arrangement and even their polarities.

In addition, every pyramid contained an orb of energy that spun clockwise, mimicking the circular motion of the spiral. Each orb contained the highest frequencies of color, light, and sound within the heart of the pyramid. In fact, the orbs became the living containment of the original source energy. As it rotated, the source energy acted much like a gyroscope, maintaining balance within each pyramid.

The Formation of Matter

Later, the pyramids began to further organize into larger particles that ultimately became octahedrons. These looked like balls of energy with flat areas on the outside. Each octahedron contained the individual consciousness of each of its inner pyramids as well as the consciousness of itself as a separate manifested aspect of creation. Consciousness within formed matter had become more complex.

In time, the octahedrons began to organize based upon their inner polarities. They aligned based upon opposite polarities in the same way that magnets of opposite poles will back up from each other. As the octahedrons aligned based upon these opposite polarities, what occurred were empty spaces between each particle.

This arrangement of particles and spaces became the basic layout of all creation. Manifested Creation became particles of living light and consciousness that arranged themselves to create actual matter and levels of reality. And within every layer and aspect of this structure of creation, every particle retained its singular and collective consciousness.

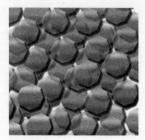

Particulates arranging to form matter.

Within these spaces, conscious energy began to flow. As the energy flowed through the tiny corridors, it collected memories of all of its experiences and communicated that information to every octahedron particle it passed. When the energy communicated to the particulates, they began to rearrange and create new forms of matter, which became new and different aspects of reality.

As new and different reality came to life, so did layers of reality in the form of dimensional arrangements. At the very center of creation, a sphere of source light remained in exactly the same frequency and manner that was formed in the center of each basic pyramid. Immediately beyond its center was a void, a level of nothingness except for dark matter that continued to pulse and move rhythmically. From there, each consecutive layer of reality beginning first in the form of extreme density became lighter and lighter at each level of creation. The farther out from the center of creation, the lighter the layer of reality became.

All levels of reality formed into dimensions of consciousness that ultimately became alive with manifested beings of consciousness. Following the basic pattern of construct, the dimensions formed in exactly the same shape and manner of alignment as the basic octahedronal particles had at the beginning of the process. As the dimensions aligned one above the other, the energy within them continued to move in spiral fashion just as the original fragments of light had done.

The inner dimensions, because of their extreme density, contained no organized life. Moving away from the dense core, as the organizational structure and the consciousness within it became less and less restricted by the weight of creation, lighter and lighter beings of different combinations of frequencies and density also formed.

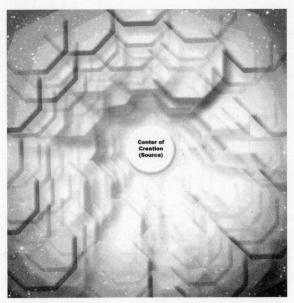

Dimensional reality is formed.

The deeper dimensions became the breeding ground for dark beings, those of base natures and no real memory of the beginning. Their motivations were based strictly upon themselves, and they became parasites, sucking the energy out of everything around them in order to survive. They were the first true parasites in creation, and they were an extremely primitive aspect of consciousness. They became violent and aggressive, but during that time, generally remained in their respective layers of reality.

The more central areas of reality contained the third, fourth, and fifth dimensions as well as the astral planes. It is in these areas that great emotion grew unrestricted, and undefined consciousness came into being as well as, later, humanity and other creatures great and small.

Outward still came the dimensions of the sixth, seventh, and eighth, highly mental dimensions with not only the memory of all time but the awareness of it. In these dimensions there was little emotion as all events past, present, and future, continually recorded the experiences of the inner planes and those above it.

Beyond the mental came the causal planes, beginning with the tenth-dimensional plane. This level of reality became the bridge point between the first through the ninth planes of reality and the eleventh and twelfth planes of being. The tenth plane was a harmonic octave point, capable of morphing its reality and the very consciousness within it in order to maintain the balance between the inner and outer worlds.

The areas of the eleventh and twelfth planes became the highest of high, composed of the most similar frequencies relative to the original source. There, disembodied forms of consciousness become a reality, and due to their lack of density, they became able to travel freely amongst the planes. They became the watchers and the Masters, the guides and teachers of all other manifested creatures.

Beyond the dimension of the twelfth there was again light, a field of energy remnant from the original source, blinding in its perfection. The outer source level's containment of all aspects of reality was also a cohesive field of consciousness that held awareness of the totality with no aspect of individuality.

The Inner and Outer Corridors of Creation

In the same way that the corridors of flowing energy remained between the original octahedronal particulates, corridors also remained between all of the dimensional layers. Because of the spiral movement and pulsation of this highly organized mass of creation, the corridors occasionally overlapped, opening avenues between worlds and dimensions. These avenues ultimately became inter-dimensional portals that opened and closed as alignments came and went and the movement continued. The corridors also linked occasionally in the overall movement to form what we now call star gates and wormholes. Wormholes are shortcuts in the fabric of creation. Star gates are the doorways between the various areas of wormholes.

Between every particulate and each dimensional level of reality, the perimeters are angulated. The angulations on the edges of the particulates and dimensions remain constant, repetitive, no matter how large or small reality has manifested. No matter what direction or level of reality, these angles are consistently divisible by fifteen degrees.

Angulations between the dimensions became pathways for energy and consciousness as well as for inter-galactic travelers to access the dimensional doorways, or portals. In the corridors of the minuscule particulate arrangements, the angulations were identical to those that had formed in the vast and infinite corridors of organized dimensional reality.

Within the tiny pathways between octahedronal particulates, energy flows constantly. The energy contained information and, later, prayers, and intentions. As the energies move through the vast corridors of creation, they communicate information, memories, and instructions. The various layers of reality were informed about what was going on throughout creation. They were told what still needed to be created, what no longer worked, and the general needs within each aspect of reality, as well as virtually anything and everything that happened.

This entire process continues even now. When the energies pass by and between particulates, the particulates receive instructions and in response rearrange in their respective places and create a new reality. They might turn slightly, or they may at times even roll over in place. As each particulate changes position, new and different alignments occur with every surrounding particulate. When the new arrangement is complete, a new reality is formed. This is how our prayers are answered, how miracles happen, and how generally what we intend comes to fruition.

Sometimes a new reality forms immediately, while at other times the particulates begin to kind of wobble in place, but a new reality isn't quite created, or the outcome is a lesser version of reality and perhaps even a less desirable one. This is because the instructions contained within the energy were not clear to begin with. There are many reasons for that, but in terms of creating new or different realities when we are attempting to manifest an outcome, or in the case of energy healing, it is because our intentions were not made clear to begin with.

Using Our Consciousness to Change Reality

Because of the way matter is naturally created within the overall organizational structure of creation, every particle that we are created of carries the light of the source. We are literally filled with memories and knowledge of everything that has ever been. Our consciousness is the energy that connects the dots of all of the particles within us as we access the different levels of Gamma Consciousness.

This is how ascension works. When we move into gamma state, all of the particles in our bodies become unified by the expansion of the tiny energy fields of our DNA strands. As these little energy fields expand, they begin to connect to each other. As they do, our bodies, minds, and spirits are unified, and we are consciously part of creation and intentionally merging our consciousness with our source.

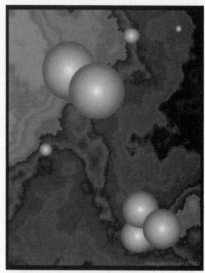

Our intention with doubts, fears, negative beliefs.

When we are intentionally connected within the construct of creation through our higher forms of conscious awareness, we intentionally expand the light within us to harmonize with the light of the source that is within all aspects of creation. Because we are created in exactly the same process as the rest of reality, each of us is unique in our overall harmonization. At the same time, we are inter-linked with the pathways of creation just like the notes of a vast musical chord form part of a greater harmonic whole.

Even when we are not in ascension mode, part of our inherent make-up is always aware of what is happening universally. That part is our infinite consciousness. This constant awareness is within us and all around us, and not ever part of our logical thinking selves. In fact, when our thinking mind is active and the neurons are firing as the logic of our thoughts progress, the electrical zapping that is going on in our brains actually closes the doors to our infinite consciousness.

When we enter into our Seventh Sense, our logical minds quiet down, the electrical impulses slow, operating at a minimum, and we are able to reconnect our consciousness and, therefore, our awareness throughout our bodies as well as in an unlimited fashion into the universal consciousness. It is at this point when we can create reality that shows up instantaneously. We can also connect with the energy body of another being to merge into a universal state of consciousness to effect healing. In addition, we can exchange information with others in the same format.

How to Effectively Make New Reality

Using our consciousness on specific levels, creating a new reality or specific outcomes is quite simple. Instead of focusing on the process, we focus on the outcome. Not the details, not ever. Instead, we focus on the emotions and sensations of how we will feel when we have reached the outcome of our intended reality. If we focus on the details or our negative emotions about what we want to create, we send the messages out in a way that is not cohesive or strong in its request and, instead, nothing happens or, worse, we witness the beginning of our manifestation in reality as it begins to create, and then things happen to stop the process.

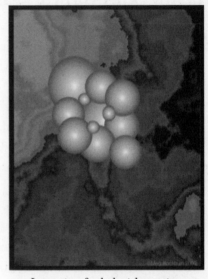

Intention fueled with passion

To create a reality effectively we must imagine the outcome with all of our senses and emotions. Breathe that reality into our bodies and then, as if we are throwing an Etheric ball, release the intention of that reality out into the universal process and fuel it with the emotions from our heart space. Then, we have sent clear unhindered intentions with a definite outcome into the creative process. In sending the intentions out so purely what we have done is left the details up to creation. In doing so, we have not limited the outcome to only the details we might have listed, but instead, we have asked creation to provide our new reality from the infinite possibilities that are available. Usually the outcome is even better than we could have imagined it and comes much faster because there are no details holding it back.

Once the intention is released into the creative process, there is no reason whatsoever to repeat it. Why? Because each time it is repeated, our state of mind, body, and spirit is different. So are our feelings. This is why affirmations don't really work and why it isn't a good idea to repeat a thought or intention over and over again. When we do, we send the same signal out over and over again with slightly different instructions.

Mergence with Another Person, Group, or Any Other Form of Reality

Much in the same way that we create new realities for ourselves, we can merge with the consciousness of another person, creature, or object. In this case, we are not projecting an intention. Instead, we are projecting our attention in the form of our conscious awareness.

In multi-dimensional healing, the healer literally merges his or her consciousness within the energy field of the other person. At this point, the two are joined into one field of energy and anything can happen. Mergence with the field of another person is a huge responsibility and the most powerful form of access and healing that there is.

To understand how this happens, we must backtrack for just a minute. Remember when we did the exercise, Movement to Spirit? How the energy in our hands was our focus? That energy is also our life force, the consciousness within us. If you noticed while you were focused upon the energy between your hands during the exercise, you might have also noticed that that energy was actually a ball shape. When we do that exercise and expand the energy between our hands, it becomes a rotating sphere of energy just like the center of creation. Just like the center of the pyramid. Just like creation in action.

Merging with the field of another person is a very powerful thing to do. It requires impeccable integrity and care. When in practice, this tool does not obviously seem to be a big deal but whatever we think, emote, or intend, in fact, anything that goes through any part of us also goes to the person who is in our hands. The other person's field will quickly respond to the instructions that flow through us even if those instructions were not meant to be given and were an unintentional thought we had, an imagining, or anything, so we need to be perfectly clear that this isn't just something cool to do. Mergence with the field of another being is a powerful tool for teaching, healing, and reading the energy field of another.

Exercise Two: Field Mergence

A perfect way to easily learn to merge with the field of another person is to first bring up the energy in your hands. Close your eyes and focus on that energy and breathe. Let the energy expand between your hands until you feel like it has become an orb and stabilized into a reasonably strong force.

Once the sphere is achieved, move your hands (while still holding the sphere of energy) to either side of your client's head and be still. Focus only on the energy between your hands. What happens next is amazing. You may begin to feel a slight shift in the energy as if it is sliding or rocking between your hands, or you might feel a slight bump. You might feel like the energy has just doubled in size or has sped up. You might feel all three of these things or none of them.

When you bring the sphere of your life force, your living consciousness, into the head of your client, your client's life force recognizes the source energy in the sphere, and the client's consciousness creates a similar sphere that reaches out and merges with the energy in your hands. When this takes place, your energy field and that of your client are completely merged. As long as you remain connected, the two of you are sharing energy fields in tandem.

In this type of mergence, transmutation of energy can be done. So can transfer of information. Healing of different areas of the energy field can occur. In fact, nothing that is intended can't be done. We will explore these things more later.

The most important caveat that I can give to the reader at this point is to remember that energy transfers. If we as healers have not dealt with our own issues, if we are insecure or not generally clear of our fears, issues,

Continued

and other negative things, the energy of any or all of those things can and may transfer into our client.

Do not at any time, ever, connect with another person with any intention made or imagined. Once this powerful connection is made, whatever you intend can come quickly into reality because you have instilled its energy into the other person's Etheric field. I can't stress enough how powerful this connection is and the damage that can be done by wayward thought, emotions, and intentions!

In the same way our stuff transfers to the client, what the client has in his or her energy field can transfer into us. We must be diligent about taking care of ourselves first as beings of creation as well as to establish protection before making the mergence connection. Once that protection is established, nothing can get through the protective field.

Exercise Three: Establishing Etheric Protection

Before we work in states of higher consciousness or we become merged within the energy field of another person, and before we open ourselves to become exposed to their energies and all that may affect them, it is paramount that we establish a protective field so that we are not vulnerable to otherworldly influences. Also, as I have mentioned before, energy transfers. Not just specific types of energy, all energy.

Many people believe that using tools that surround us with energy creating a protective bubble around us is enough. Others believe that surrounding ourselves with mirrors is all we need. Let's change our perception to consider that we have already learned that we are everything and everything is created of us. Therefore what we encounter within other worlds also lives within us.

There is only one way to go about self-protection that is impenetrable and completely safe in every circumstance and that is using the source light within us.

Here is how to make that happen:

Close your eyes and focus your attention to the very center of your being. It will seem very dark at first as if there is nothing in there. Project your attention further inside of yourself, down to your very core. There you will see or sense a tiny little light that is light golden white in color. If you don't see ethereally, you may sense a tiny warm spot.

Once you locate the little light or warm place, begin to breathe, directing your breath into the light. Notice that with each breath that you project into this light, the light and its warmth grow larger and larger. Keep breathing.

Eventually, the light will have filled your body and begun to overflow around the outside of your body. Keep breathing into the light until it has created an elliptic (oval) field of light around you. The light will organize into this elliptic shape on its own. Once the light field has stabilized and you feel that you have achieved being completely surrounded by a field of this energy, intend for it to remain in place. It will.

The protective field that you have created is made out of the source light from within your particulates. Nothing of any less frequency or vibration less than the pure vibration of the source can enter into that field—no energy, no kind of being of any kind, nothing.

This exercise is good to do every morning before you even get out of bed so that you are protected from picking up unwanted energies when you are out and about. Sometimes when we encounter people in our daily errands, they have very strong motivations or intentions that are not necessarily good for us to take into our personal energy fields. Some people tend to force their energy outward and into others when they are trying to make a point. When this source field is up and active, no one can force their energy into your field intentionally or otherwise.

Exercise Four: Transferring Information from the Akashic Records

In the same way that we can project our energy in the form of consciousness into our hands and into a mergence with the energy field of another person, we can also project our consciousness by using our energy field and raising it upward through our crown.

Doing this is a lot like raising invisible antennae to connect within the universal memory, also known as the Akashic records. The Akashic records are not found only on one level of creation or in some secret room out there in the universe somewhere; the information of all time is stored in every tiny particle of creation. Raising our consciousness up beyond our crown and above our personal Etheric field is an intentional connection into the fabric of creation so that it can tell us whatever we want to know. Making this connection is not hard at all once you stop thinking about how it works.

To receive information, it is best to formulate your question before doing this exercise. Once you get the hang of it you will learn to imagine your question and raise your Etheric antennae simultaneously. It just takes practice. An easy way to get your antennae up and running is to again go back to that ball of conscious energy you have learned how to make between your hands. This time, instead of connecting with someone else, bring the energy up to your head, just like you learned how to do when connecting with the head of another person. First, hold the orb above your head; then when you begin to feel something change, gently and slowly bring the orb down into your head and imagine that the orb is stretching upward through the crown of your head and into the heavens.

Once you have projected your energy upward, making your Etheric connection, imagine that it begins to spread out and seems to dissipate into the empty spaces between the particulates (the little octahedrons that organized to create matter). Don't be specific about where your energy goes; just imagine that it is running through whatever passages it finds. Believe it or not, this conscious energy knows where to go, what to do, how to do it, and where it needs to flow without any specific instructions *from you. Once connected, information is everywhere in everything so the where doesn't matter.*

In the same way that the energy of your consciousness flows in the corridors of creation, the answers you seek will flow into your request. The important thing here is not to expect what the answer will be or what the experience will be like. It will come, if you have gotten out of the way. Answers come very differently using this form of awareness. They don't come as logically stated information. They come in a variety of ways. They might come as pictures, little movies, feelings, or knowings.

However it comes for you, the information becomes a permanent part of you, stored in your light field until you need it.

If you begin to sense that you are receiving an answer, and you start to logically think about that answer to try to understand it, you will immediately close the connection that you had opened. Sometimes information comes in pieces or fragments and doesn't seem to make sense. Because the information isn't linear like information is in our brains, this is a new way of comprehending. In this new way, we are receiving information holographically. When information moves within the construct of creation, the information is carried in and reflected by light. The information comes into us as pure light energy so our logical brains can't translate it. It literally becomes part of us and will surface as we need it. The fragments will come together at the exact moment we need the information, and with a little relaxation, both the information flow and its translation become much more efficient with practice.

Remote Viewing, Long Distance Healing, and Traveling Inter-Dimensionally in Time and Space

Once we become more proficient at projecting our consciousness to connect with another or to gain information for specific reasons, we can progress to projecting in more general ways in order to access distant people or places and even times.

In the same way our intentions and prayers move through the most min-ute pathways and corridors of reality, our consciousness can travel through the inter-dimensional corridors beyond time and space, across dimensional barriers (some like to call these the "veils") and into specific locales both here on earth and in completely new and different levels of reality. These corridors function in exactly the same way as energy traveling on a particulate level, but in this case it is intentional consciousness with a purpose that is traveling the larger corridors between dimensions.

Believe it or not, all time, past, present, and future is occurring simultane-ously because of the way creation remembers everything. As it remembers, cre-ation also begins to organize toward possible outcomes. As outcomes begin to form, more possibilities are created. In every moment that we exist, the future is already in motion. So is the past.

The best place to be among all of this confusing memory is right now. Noth-ing ever happens outside of a now. What has been continues to exist as indelible memories in a field of light. What is not yet created is an intricately woven set of universal actions and reactions that has not yet taken form.

Remote viewing is nothing more than allowing yourself to relax enough to let your consciousness stretch to a specific destination for a specific reason. It can be fun too. Once you have learned to project your consciousness at will, you can send your consciousness anywhere you want it to go.

As I experienced different levels of consciousness, I actually began doing this spontaneously. I had no idea how it worked or why or how to do it on purpose and so had to backtrack how it worked. Remote viewing came in very handy with my best friend. We had known each other for nearly 30 years and during that time no matter how close or far we lived from each other, we had coffee together either in person or over the phone.

I tend to be an early bird and was often awake before my friend, so I began to "check in" on her before ringing her up on the phone. Careful to respect her pri-vacy, I always aimed my remote sight for her hands and coffee mug. If I saw them together, I knew she was up and active. If I saw one and not the other, I waited until a little later to call.

Besides being a fun everyday tool, remote viewing has been used for much more serious things. Certain factions of different governments have taught, or attempted to teach, groups of civilians and soldiers how to remote view as an experiment toward, shall we say, knowing what the enemy is up to.

Remote viewing really isn't hard to learn and can be very useful when checking on your children, loved ones, etc. Privacy issues do apply in remote viewing, so courtesy needs to be considered.

Remote healing works similarly. In order to locate the client or subject (some people like to work on locations as well as people) simply imagine them and let your consciousness rise up through your crown and go. Your consciousness already recognizes your target and will link up almost immediately.

Traveling inter-dimensionally can be so much less specific than remote viewing or healing, as most of the time we don't consciously know our way around creation, but there are roadmaps encoded within us. I have found it to be the most beneficial to let my consciousness free flow dimensionally. The experiences are always much fuller and vivid, and I have learned an immense amount by trusting the process. If an experience begins that needs to continue, and we need to disrupt it due to time or place restraints in our 3-D world, we can immediately return to where we were even mid-sentence, if talking with a being in another world, simply by intending to pick up where we left off.

A great example of how this works from the "other side" is when I channel private sessions for clients on occasion. The Masters and I have established such a beautiful relationship and they are so helpful, I occasionally let them use my body to talk to people who don't know how to communicate with them any other way.

Typically, these sessions are done over the phone. Time and again, it has amazed people when for some reason the session is interrupted. The Masters' energy is very intense and often drains phone batteries or messes with our phone connections or with electronics in general. When the connection is lost and we reconnect the call, the Masters pick up mid-sentence right *exactly* where they left off without a pause or a glitch as if no time has passed at all. It is as if there was never an interruption. That is because they are not limited by time or space, and it is simply our attention that temporarily left. They never leave. This is hard to understand but, on the other hand, makes perfect sense. We are the ones with perceived limitations, and by our perceptions, the limitations are created.

Exercise Five: Intentional Out of Body Travel

Due to the nature of this exercise, some safety issues must be established. Before beginning this exercise, there are a few very important things that you must do.

- *First, make yourself a promise that no matter what happens you are having your own experience, you are in control, and if you become uncomfortable at any time you can simply stop doing it.*

- *Promise yourself that no matter where you find your consciousness you will return to your body when you are finished with your experience.*

- *No exceptions.*

The reason that it is necessary to set some safety terms for yourself up front is that the levels of consciousness you are learning here are unlimited in scope and possibility. Anything can happen, and, frankly, once you find the on switch to this kind of being, it is very difficult to want to turn it off. In fact, out of body inter-dimensional travel can be downright addictive.

Some of the places or feelings that you may experience can be so bliss-ful that you just want to stay "out there" forever. That is not okay. You are a human being, having come to the earth for a multitude of reasons, but that is another story for another time. The point is that you are here for a journey that you have committed to take and you must finish that journey not by leaping out of your body and skipping all the good parts!

One of the best ways to become really present before beginning this exercise is to begin to notice everything around you and every detail of every thing. Look at your hands. Look at your feet. Take some slow, delib-erate breaths and, as you do, listen to your breath. Listen to your breath again. Continue listening to your breath, and close your eyes. The more present you can bring yourself, the greater your freedom becomes out of body because fewer distractions are holding you back.

Once you are fully present and in your body completely, start to raise your Etheric antennae. Let your energy rise up and out of your crown, and then let it go. Really, just let it go. No matter what, your consciousness remains attached to your main field. As it moves away from your body, the connection between your consciousness and body stretches like an invisible rubber band. Knowing that this connection remains in place takes a lot of the possible fear factor out of the situation. Be still, don't think, don't worry about what is or isn't happening; focus on the energy as it rises up through your crown and begins to seek experiences on its own, and see what happens. It is best not to give yourself specific target times or destinations until you become proficient with the sensations, energy shifts, and reality challenges that can come with these kinds of experiences. It will likely be very difficult at first for you to maintain your connection anywhere, so let your consciousness wander and find its way.

The impressions that you begin to get are from your consciousness traveling outside of your body, so your impressions may not make a lot of sense at first. The more you do this exercise, the greater expansion your awareness will have.

If you try this method of achieving a connection consciously and it isn't working for you, chances are that you are trying too hard, have expectations that are not realistic or are limiting your experience, or maybe even some fear of the unknown has crept in. The greatest emotional place that you can use to move into multi-dimensional reality is pure humility. When the ego and the thinking selves come together, we don't stand a chance of going anywhere because we think we are in control. It can be difficult to let go of control enough to give yourself this freedom, but it is worth doing so that you can have the kinds of experiences that are available to you.

An easy way to safely achieve inter-dimensional out of body experience is to work within the sacred geometry format. Using the four-sided Pyramids, you can safely allow your consciousness to leave your body while you keep it safe inside the container of the pyramid.

Exercise Six: The Pyramid and Multi-Dimensional Awareness

Now that we have a good feel for consciousness and its possibilities, let's learn how to go multi-dimensional. Remember, the Pyramid is the most basic form of constructed reality. Using this form is the safest and easiest way to experience multi-dimensional reality for the first time.

Since the pyramid is an actual part of creation, whatever you imagine while inside of it can create so be careful what is in or on your mind when entering this exercise. I usually suggest that if you are having any kind of a challenging day or you are worried or angry, wait until your feelings change before attempting this exercise.

Step One—The Upright Pyramid

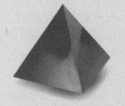

It is important to enter this series of exercises without expectations or intent. These exercises are simply for understanding your connection as a purer consciousness within the Universal process. During this exercise, you can use the four-sided pyramid to experience yourself outside of the denseness of your body. By doing so, you will begin to understand yourself as an essence that is quite separate and different from the body that you presently inhabit.

It is best to do these exercises in the order that they are given both for the quality of the experience and the fullness of your understanding. Skipping ahead does not mean that you will learn this faster—only that you will have lots of pieces of information that don't yet fit together to make sense.

To begin, close your eyes and imagine a pyramid that is created of Light. It has no density. The Light is a golden yellow and the form of the pyramid is composed of millions of tiny little dots of that Light. (If you can't quite picture a pyramid, start by imagining a triangle). The pyramid is four sided, and larger than your body. Imagine that this pyramid is floating in front of you and that you can step inside of it. This pyramid that you have envisioned is a hologram.

When you feel comfortable with this image, imagine that you are step-ping inside of the pyramid. Once you have stepped inside, imagine that you are sitting down inside of the pyramid.

Once you are inside of the pyramid, one of the first things that you will notice is that you feel free and light. The air you are breathing may begin to feel cold in your nostrils, and you may hear or feel a slight but consistent hum. The tone of the hum that you are hearing is your unique harmonic sig-nature. The tone, or hum, may seem to have a pulsing from deep within your perception. Your tongue will automatically move to the roof of your mouth.

Experience this feeling. Notice what it feels like to be free of your body. Notice that the energy in your body has become different and that you feel very connected to everything at once, yet you remain aware of yourself. You may have other visual or aural experiences during this exercise.

(It is important to note that you are always in control of your experi-ence. If at any time you begin to feel uncomfortable in any way, simply stop the exercise.)

Experience the feeling within the pyramid as long as you are comfort-able and able to maintain the exercise. Then simply desire to return to your physical body. Notice how you feel . . . clearer, lighter, and freer. Balanced and more in touch.

Congratulations! You have just taken your first step into multi-dimensional awareness!

If you wish, do this exercise for a week or more until you feel very comfortable with the energies and the experience. If it helps, take notes to track your progress. Gaining a large degree of comfort within the pyramid will assist you in the next phases of the exercises.

Step Two—The Inverted Pyramid

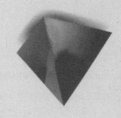

Now that you have experienced yourself as pure consciousness in the form of an upright four-sided pyramid, you can progress into the Universal per-spective. To do this, close your eyes and picture the

Continued

same kind of pyramid (or triangle) that you worked with in the previous exercise and, with your imagination, turn it upside down.

The pyramid now looks much like a V, or a satellite dish, a receiver of sorts. Once you have obtained this image and it feels comfortable to you, use your consciousness to step into the inverted pyramid (this may be a bit more difficult than the first exercise until you have practiced a bit because the energy within the inverted pyramid is quite different than what you experienced during the first exercise).

Having stepped into the inverted pyramid, you have intentionally joined the Universal consciousness.

Allow yourself to sit with these new energies. What do you hear? What do you feel? With your ethereal eyes, what do you see? Each of you will have your own experience with this part of the exercise because you are each made of different sets of frequencies. How your awareness perceives this experience is based upon what frequencies you carry within you.

It takes longer for some to understand the information they receive in the inverted pyramid while others who work with this exercise will quickly understand. Since there is no competition "out there" beyond the third-dimensional reality, it really doesn't matter how long it takes you to "get it." With practice the information will come and the experience will broaden.

Some of the information you receive while in this inverted pyramid may be in conceptual form, while other information may come to you with fine details. It is important not to think about what you are receiving—just let yourself receive. In the moments that you are doing this exercise, you have joined the Universal process in real time. You, in those moments, are intentionally receiving information via the null zones of the universal construct that is communicating to your personal particulates. You are intentionally being a part of the information flow throughout all things. You have become the moment.

Do this exercise, if you wish, for about a week or until you feel that you have mastered consciousness from within the inverted pyramid. Pay close attention to your perceptions during this part of the exercise as they will be quite different than those of week one.

Step Three—Putting It All Together

Now you have experienced yourself both as pure consciousness and as an intentional member of the consciousness of the One. This exercise will teach you to pull yourself together on Universal terms . . . with a few surprises.

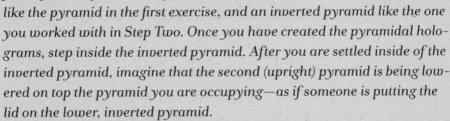

To do this part of the exercise, you must close your eyes and picture two pyramids—one upright, like the pyramid in the first exercise, and an inverted pyramid like the one you worked with in Step Two. Once you have created the pyramidal holograms, step inside the inverted pyramid. After you are settled inside of the inverted pyramid, imagine that the second (upright) pyramid is being lowered on top the pyramid you are occupying—as if someone is putting the lid on the lower, inverted pyramid.

As the upright pyramid is lowered onto you while you are within the inverted pyramid, ask the upright pyramid to turn forty-five degrees so that the corners of the upright and the inverted pyramids form a star on the exterior. Lower the upper pyramid down two thirds of the way over yourself within the inverted pyramid.

You now have a complete representation of yourself as a conscious being within the Universal perspective. You may begin to hear your harmonic signature again.

In a different environment, such as another planet or dimension, this tone or combination of tones would sound different to you. This has to do with local environmental harmonic resonance.

The energy that you feel while you occupy this geometric formation is quite powerful. It is as if you are in the middle of all creation. You are. As mentioned earlier, within each pyramid resides a sphere of energy.

Continued

That energy represents perfection just as it did within the formation of the holographic pyramids that ultimately became the particulates. Of course, when you are working with holograms, the spheres within the pyramids become holographic too. They have shape and dimension, and they spin.

As the two pyramids join—one upright, one inverted—the spherical energies within the pyramids are spinning. As they are placed one on top of the other, the spheres—now globes of spinning energy—begin to flatten out. For a short while, from a side view, the flattening circles begin to look like an infinity sign (an eight on its side). The energies of the two circles wobble briefly as the two come together, and then in an instant they open up together, releasing the perfect energy that has been held within their centers.

Interpreting Your Experiences

When we begin to access multi-dimensional awareness, our sense of reality can be challenged to the max. Our value system begins to lose some of the stringent beliefs we had carried before. When we begin to experience how subtle and intricate, how fragile, how powerful, and how miraculous creation is and how our consciousness links in with creation, it is really difficult to hold onto stubborn beliefs that never really served us anyway. We begin to realize that everything is truly small stuff and nothing is worth the drama and trauma that we had allowed in life previous to our new understandings.

We also begin to realize how effortlessly we can change our life experience and that the old ways of struggling to achieve an outcome were a real waste of time.

But how do we know what the new experiences are telling us? How do we know what is important and what isn't? Like opening a new pair of eyes that has never witnessed our world, changing states of consciousness come with a lot of questions that can't be answered any other way than by having the experience.

The worst thing to do when beginning to enter into altered reality is to let the imagination out to play while interpreting the meanings of our encounters.

Seriously. I see so many people try to apply a familiar name to something just to feel as if they have achieved something. This can cause their experiences to go from what started as real to a complete fantasy. Not every being on the other side is named Quan Yin or Archangel Michael or Mary Magdalene or . . . well, hopefully you get my point. Not that some people aren't in touch with these Masters; they are. It is just that people in general tend to name names that they know in order to make sense of their experience, or for the energy that is coming through to be conveyed as powerfully as it might feel to them.

Often the guide or Master who is giving assistance doesn't have a name that is even pronounceable in our language. When we access layers of reality that are far beyond what we know, everything consists of pure harmonic resonance, combinations of tones that resonate within creation. This includes language too. The far out harmonics are composed of tones and combinations of tones that are extremely high frequency and may not be audible in our aural spectrum. The harmonics cannot always be translated into words. Besides, in our current languages, words define completely and leave no room for subtleties that can add meaning to an experience. Some of the more ancient languages we have had on earth were based upon inference of subtleties in their expression. Those languages were closer to truth than our current ones.

There is an emotional place inside of us that comes with these experiences that feels so holy that we instinctively want to reach outward in order to understand it. Because of this, we tend to want to name our experiences based upon something familiar.

Nope. Not. Don't do it. If you are not given a name, just let it be what it is. Sometimes there is more truth in the not defining.

Labels are not important and don't mean anything to anyone but us anyway. The important thing to remember is: how does the experience feel? Does it feel true? Does it give you an insight? Do you feel comfortable with what happened? Yes? Go for it. Find out more. No? Why not? What wasn't comfortable about it? Did where you were or the life form you were with during your experience feel heavy or like something you didn't want to trust? Chances are you were right. Did the information you were receiving feel like truth or not? Find out by asking yourself what was not comfortable for you. Usually this is because at first the experiences are new and don't really seem to have any real parameters for comparison, so there is no frame of reference in place from which we can create a comfort zone.

The best way to interpret the real meaning, if any, of these new experiences is by looking first at the symbolism. Were there objects, shapes, colors, or people who mean specific things to you? If so, what do they mean? Start with the most obvious; then move to the less obvious. The greatest advice I can give you on interpretation is to trust your guts.

The more you think about your experiences, the less true they become.

Maybe you are receiving fragments of information or flashes at first; perhaps you notice a flash of color (this is normal and usually the first clue that you are using your third eye). What does that color mean to you? Don't know? Okay, how does it make you *feel*? When you think of that color what happens *inside* of you?

Basically, no two people perceive anything exactly the same way. We perceive not only with our five senses, but with our sixth and seventh senses as well. Some of us see moving pictures in our heads as if a movie were playing out. Others see still pictures, or a combination of moving and still. Some people don't see at all, and that is fine too. Some people feel things inside of them and factor their experiences by the nature of that feeling. Others just know. Even others have an entire set of skills and get a whole body knowing with pictures, sound, and feelings. No matter what your way of sensing is, just remember that we are all capable of tapping into extended reality and comprehending exactly what we need if we choose.

Something else to remember when we send our consciousness into extended reality is to pay attention to our surroundings. You can learn a lot by being aware of what is around you when you are out of body. To me, being out of body looks like a very different version of our world. All of my senses remain active while I have the experience. Of course, it wasn't always like that; time and practice brought on new and different attributes to my gifts.

But seriously, pay attention.

I was in Peru for special ceremonies with some close friends who are indigenous Incan people. Several groups were in attendance, and during the journey, we went across Lake Titicaca to the Isle of Amantani to spend the night with the people there. It is a magical place with many legends and myths about mermaids and cities under the lake. Almost as soon as we arrived on the island, my sense of reality began to shift, and I began to have profound visions of underwater caves, caves that were partly submerged, and rooms that were carved out of rock and had ancient writing carved all over the ceilings. I was spontaneously remote viewing but honestly wasn't sure *where* I was seeing or *when*. That can happen. Anyway, I let my visions wander through the caves and I found myself seeing them from different angles, different areas, and even different elevations. I looked around carefully for something that would help me identify where I was should the opportunity come up that I could discuss the visions with someone local who might know. Looking for landmarks or some sort of identity markers is always a good thing.

The next day a woman I had never met from one of the other groups approached me and said that she and her friend were both having profound visions of underwater caves and rooms. Her description up to that moment was identical to what I had been seeing. I began to question her about details, trying to validate the connection. It can be extremely meaningful when multiple people have the same experiences simultaneously, especially when they don't know each other.

As I asked her for details, I started to ask about the ancient writing I had seen, and about some other minor details I had picked up on. She wanted to know where I had seen the writing, and I told her on the ceiling. "Gee," she said, "I never thought to look up!"

We can miss a lot because we are overwhelmed with the power of these experiences when we are having them. We don't have to chronicle every detail, but I have learned that consciousness goes to where the most important information of the moment is, even when we don't realize its importance. When I asked my shaman friend later about the cave system, he told me there were stories of all kinds about the caves and a civilization that is now underwater, but no one had located it yet. None of the three of us who had the visions had ever heard any of those stories. My sense was that the caves were extremely near where we stayed on the island; they may even have been underneath us. That three of us who didn't know each other had nearly identical visions was no coincidence.

One of the rules that I use to validate my experiences is that if information, signs, signposts, anything comes in threes, there is truth to it. In other words, three people having the same visions, hearing the same name, word, or subject three times in a short period of time, all of these things indicate a truth that we really need to pay attention to.

One of my favorite stories about things coming in threes is how listening to those signs changed the course of my life practically overnight. Sometimes when the Masters attempt to guide me in a certain direction, I resist out of stubbornness, or I may be busy and ignore them. Honestly, being "online" 24/7 can get annoying sometimes!

Shortly after my huge awakening and embracing my paranormal gifts and learning to put them to positive use, I met my husband. We became very involved, and before we got married, his company transferred him across the country. He was transferred with no notice and on his way out of town called and asked me to follow. About a week later I did. I was in a place that was strange to me, three thousand miles from home, and had been there for about a week. I have to admit that I was feeling kind of homesick. My new guy had gone to work, and there I was stuck in a hotel room in a strange place trying to figure out what to do next. Having just left my very busy private practice, I had no idea what I would do for work or where to start.

Before I left North Carolina, I had a weekly meeting with a group of people who met in my home while I channeled the Masters. The group started every Wednesday evening at seven and without fail the Masters would express their presence through me. Often the Masters were so excited about something they had to share that night, they would try to come through even earlier, and I would have to hold them off until everyone arrived.

There I was alone in the hotel room, and right at 4:00 p.m. Pacific Time (7:00 p.m. Eastern Time), the Masters started talking in my head. I laughed and said aloud to them, "Sorry, but no one is here but you and me." And they started talking again.

For the second time, I said, a little more loudly and with more effort, "Listen, guys, there isn't anyone here but you and me." And a third time, they started talking again.

How annoying. They can be that way when they have something important for me to hear. In protest, I swept my arm around the hotel room and said to them (I must have looked ridiculous since I was the only visible "person" there), "Will you *please* listen to me? Look around! There is *you* and *me* and we have *no audience!*"

"Yes we do," they said smugly. "*You* have a *computer!*" Oh my God. They were right. I had brought my laptop. Okay. They won that round. I sat down and started typing what they said. At the time I had a whopping twenty-four people on my email list. I sent the Masters' message out to all of them. And they forwarded it. And it got forwarded again. And again. And again. By the second week, I had over 8,000 requests to join my email list. Every technology I had for email back then crashed with the sheer number of subscriptions. Ultimately, I figured out how to keep up with it all, and that was the beginning of the Online Messages. The Online Messages have spanned the globe, created a huge network of people, and instigated my website and even some of the information in my books. The Online Messages have been going on ten years and now reach an estimated quarter million people per month. They are still growing, all because someone "out there" wouldn't stop talking three different times—and I finally got the message. The whole thing was hilarious, and I am beyond grateful that I had the sense to listen.

How Consciousness Affects Our Bodies

We have learned that consciousness is pure energy. In the same way that each of us is composed of a unique formation of harmonics that comes from the arrangement of our individual sets of particulates, our consciousness is unique too. Being pure energy, consciousness is also pure harmonics. Each individual expression of consciousness consists of aspects of those harmonics.

When tones are combined, they not only include the actual notes or the sounds, but they also include what are called overtones, suggestions of, or implied, harmonics. It is in the overtones that individual consciousness comes to life. In a way, we could view this phenomenon as the highest memory bank of our individual existence.

Consciousness becomes the individual set of harmonics of the individual. Any individual consciousness can be merged with any other form of energy but cannot be duplicated. Consciousness, because we are a formed reality, remains connected within the construct of creation. We could view this as us being a living expression of our source. Man made as a reflection of God.

While we are manifested as beings of dense reality, part of us remains in the flow of the creative process and infinitely connected. It is in this way that our consciousness is constantly aware of everything that is happening within creation.

We don't usually experience this profound connection in everyday life from a cognitive state, but we do experience it in other ways. Without being really aware of our connection to our source and creation, we respond to events that occur in our world, our universe, and all of the multiverses that compose creation.

For example, when our moon is in certain stages of its rotation, like when it becomes full, we might become disturbed or emotional. Part of this reaction is the water in our bodies being pulled by gravitational forces and creating a temporary imbalance within us. Also, the water within us is conductive and carries energy through our bodies easily.

Another aspect of our reaction to a full moon is our response to the pull of gravity it creates. Gravity is the force that maintains balance in our universe. It is also a large contributing factor to the fact that our particulates hold together at all.

Gravity is a field of energy that, in a way, overlaps and is enmeshed within all forms of creation in our world. On locations where there is no gravity, there is not likely to be matter formed in the expression of living creatures. Gravity is a different set of harmonics and energy that locks the particulates in place as they come together. Consciousness is not affected by gravity at all. Consciousness, however, can affect gravity, as happens during levitation. Consciousness also has the ability to affect the arrangement of our particulates, to command change or transmutation within our individual energy fields, in order to make changes. This is what happens when we practice healing that uses our Seventh Sense. We affect the arrangement of particulates that form our reality and, therefore, our experience as human beings.

Soul Entry—How Consciousness Enters Our Bodies

How does individual consciousness get into our bodies in the first place? In order to fully explain this to you, I will share a story with you that even today remains one of the most profound experiences of my life.

I was working with a young woman and her husband who were having serious marital problems after the miscarriage of their first baby. Neither of them seemed able to fully cope with having lost their much-wanted child. The young man's mother, a nurse, had referred the couple to me in the hopes that I could help them past the problem. We had shared only a couple of sessions together up to this particular day, and this day it was the young woman's turn.

As is my practice, we talked for a while before she got on the table. She was having a hard time expressing her emotions. After a while, she hopped up on the table, and I began to work within her energy field. As I stood at her head, with my hands on either side, our fields merged. I stood there waiting for the balance of our sweet connection to complete.

All of a sudden, I felt a third presence in the room. It was standing just to my left, so close it was nearly touching me. Being used to having spirits and guides coming and going, I was surprised to notice that, "Gee, this didn't feel like one of 'mine.'" Wondering who had entered the room, I turned my head and saw an extremely bright silver blue being that was perfectly androgynous in nature. It felt exquisite, clean and clear, but a bit impatient too. It was neither male nor female, and it looked upon the young woman with what I have to describe as pure unconditional love embodied. I stood there for a moment, seeking to connect with this being in an effort to communicate with it. When I did connect, I knew instantly what was going on. Our telepathic conversation went something like this:

"You are the soul who will be the child of this woman, aren't you?"

"Yes."

"Why are you waiting? What will it take for you to enter her body and become her child?"

"I am waiting for an invitation. They (the young couple) have expressed their desire to have a child, but in their pain and disappointment they haven't actually invited me yet. They are afraid of what might happen, that I will leave like the last soul did, but I will remain."

"You don't look like you are either a male or female. Why is that?"

"It is my choice. I have been both. I have been either. In this new time, I choose to be a female child."

"What? You are planning to become this woman's baby, and you will be born as a girl?"

"Yes."

The being never took its eyes off of the young woman. I have to admit that about then I was beyond stunned. I have never met an incoming soul before, and my emotions were running rampant. I was excited. I was overwhelmed at the immensity of love the being generated. I had a million questions, and yet I had a client on my table, and I was merged with her energy field. I knew that I had to be careful of her despite my own curiosities. Tears were falling freely down my face. My client was completely out of her body.

As I continued to work, I said to the being " Obviously, I won't be around when the moment comes and you enter this body as the incoming child. Can you show me what happens? How does this work? How do you enter the body? What is it like?"

All of a sudden my reality shifted and my head was filled with a cascade of moving pictures. I watched sperm approaching an ovum. As the sperm made contact with the egg and joined it, there was an expression of energy that looked like a tiny atomic explosion. It rose up and the top of the mushroom opened like a blossoming flower. This opening was a portal, a pathway for the incoming soul's energy to enter into the newly forming embryo.

The being showed me how the energy, the consciousness of the incoming soul, free flows into the dividing cells. As the cells of the forming embryo divide over and over again, consciousness fills every one of them and is propagated cell after cell. The being showed me that consciousness becomes an integral part of mass as it forms.

It is in this way that our consciousness fills our bodies and lives within every expression of our existence. I could barely stand I was so overwhelmed with the immensity of that moment. My whole body had turned to Jell-O as I witnessed the answer to one of the most fought about questions on the planet. I continued working within the field of my client, with tears running down my face the entire time. She had fallen into an extremely relaxed state and was unaware of what was happening with me. Probably a good thing.

I began to wonder how much I should tell her. After all, I could be wrong, right? Not likely, but I am very, very careful not to give people their experiences, so to speak. She had been so devastated by her recent miscarriage that if I didn't handle this well I could make matters a whole lot worse.

But it was so real.

At the end of our session, I chatted with my client, kind of feeling her out on the subject. I didn't know her very well, and, gosh, she had been so depressed. This was a real healer's dilemma. As a human being, I wanted to shout from the rooftops that I had just learned the secret of consciousness and life, but, on the other hand, most people don't see things the way I do, and my reality can be very strange to other people.

In the end, I decided to tell my client about what had happened in a kind of edited way. I started out by asking her if she felt as if she were ready to welcome a new baby into her family. Yes, she said, without a doubt. I told her that there was a soul waiting for her invitation and that I thought it was coming very soon and would be a girl child. My client was so happy she literally floated out the door after our session.

The soul entered her body and she became with child *that day*. Exactly nine months later, my client delivered a healthy baby girl. As for me, I will carry the immensity and the beauty of that moment in me for the rest of my life.

Twins

I became so curious about what the incoming soul had shown me, I asked the Masters to show me how my new understanding related to twins. After all, there are two ways that twins usually occur. The first is that the ovum, or egg, splits into two separate zygotes usually a couple of days after the ovum is fertilized, and identical twins are formed. They are born looking alike and often having similar personalities, and a bond exists between them that has been studied by scientists for decades.

Stories abound of identical twins who are separated at birth but later meet long after they are adults, having lived similar if not identical lives. They may dress alike, have the same tastes in food, mates, friends, in fact, virtually everything. They often even marry spouses with the same names. They are empathic with each other, feeling each other's thoughts and feelings.

Identical twins often have a sixth sensory connection to the extent that each feels what is happening in the other. This can be on emotional levels as well as physical responses. Identical twins may even tell you that they do not feel whole without each other, and the death of a twin can be devastating to the remaining twin.

When the souls of identical twins enter into the portal that occurs upon conception, they enter simultaneously, briefly occupying the ovum in tandem. As the

ovum splits into what later becomes twins, each consciousness fills its respective newly forming body, but each newly formed life also retains remnants of the
other's conscious energy. The twins become fully harmonized in a synergistic
manner so that they are at once individuals, but also harmonically and indelibly
joined for the period of their lives.

Fraternal twins are different. In their case, two eggs are fertilized by two
separate sperm cells, forming two separate portals of entry. The incoming two
souls enter simultaneously, but instead of harmonizing almost as a whole in the
way that identical twins do, they harmonize opposite each other. Fraternal twins
often not only look very different, or are of opposite sex, they often have quite
opposite personalities as well. In utero, fraternal twins often harmonize together
as mirror images of each other's energy.

CHAPTER SIX

Realizing the Immensity of
Life Events beyond the Tangible

As our consciousness filters into our bodies at the time we are conceived, and our cells continue to reproduce, they carry strands of DNA within them. Each strand of DNA carries instructions to our bodies telling us what we will look like, what our personalities will be, how our bodies will react to stimulus, and myriad other sets of instructions that science has barely begun to understand.

DNA as the Mechanism of Physical Consciousness

Our DNA also carries and responds to consciousness. Each tiny DNA strand emits a field of energy that is very subtle and electromagnetic in nature. In our everyday forms of consciousness, those fields of energy remain small and seemingly insignificant. When we leap into different states of Gamma Consciousness, our DNA begins to respond by emitting a greater and greater field of energy both between the strands and around them. The higher the state of Gamma Consciousness, the larger the field becomes until, if the ascension state is realized, the fields of energy around our DNA unite throughout our bodies and we become capable of rejoining creation body, mind, and soul. Most of us don't get to that state; attaining the states of initiation and communion are more likely. When we reach either one of these high states of consciousness, the energy of our DNA

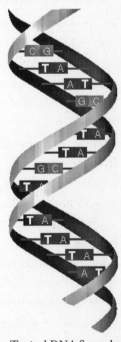

Typical DNA Strand.

strands becomes larger, and as it does, we can experience different levels of consciousness mergence.

In the same way that light records information, so does our body. Remember that as matter formed and became denser, the original source light and all of its memories were retained in every particulate. That same light continues to record our experiences and transmit that information back into creation. It also receives information from creation for us.

Also inherent in our cellular memory, our DNA, is our lineage. Everything we have ever been since the beginning of time is remembered within us. It is also remembered within our energy fields. Sometimes those memories become dense energy and cause us problems because our energy isn't flowing well. When that happens, our bodies may respond by becoming painful or sick. What we need to realize is that we are walking memory banks of, not only our entire history, but also the history of all creation.

Past Life Memory and Karma

In the same way that our particulates remember the entirety of everything that has ever happened in creation, within our energy fields are the memories of our souls. As our individual soul enters our bodies when they are mere cells dividing into a human being, all of our soul's memories are indelibly placed within the energy field. This is why some of us have fragments or even full memories of our past lives.

Past life memory usually surfaces when the memory of previous lives is applicable to our current circumstances. If we are facing a situation in our current life that is resonant with unresolved situations in our previous lifetimes, we may begin to have feelings that we can't explain, reactions that make no sense, or even experience the same situations repetitively.

When this happens, it is our history coming forward for us so that we can perhaps make different choices or resolve the situations once and for all. Unfortunately, many of us tend to resist these powerful clues and instead kick and scream our way through uncomfortable times, as we tend to resist what we don't know we want.

When those historic circumstances present themselves, part of us is asking that we resolve whatever issues are involved. This is how karma works. Experiences that we had in previous lives, or even earlier in our current lives, that we did not resolve or fully process will again present to us later on to give us the opportunity to do something different or even to learn a lesson we did not learn in the previous opportunity. We have individual karma as well as karma with other people. Karma almost always presents as a pattern of similar experiences that occur.

For example, we might find ourselves saying, "Oh, no, not again," as a certain kind of situation arises over and over again. Maybe we keep having the same kinds of painful relationships (maybe because we haven't figured out how to love ourselves and so we attract the pain from others?), or maybe we keep doing things for others only to have them stiff us somehow. (Isn't that what we have done to ourselves by giving to everyone else and not to ourselves?) Karma can show up in virtually any circumstance because it is energetically written within our energy fields.

The most powerful way to deal with karmic situations is to choose differently when a situation repeats. Making a different choice creates a different outcome and, therefore, stops the karmic pattern from happening in the future.

As healers of the Seventh Sense, we might often be shown karma within the energy field of our clients. Usually, when I see this (and we will talk more in depth about it a little later), I will stop and discuss what I have found with my client. The client will almost always recognize what I am talking about and even be eager to change the situation.

Beliefs, Fragmentation, and Our History

Hidden within the layers of our energy fields are intricate records of our life experiences. Our energy fields also record our beliefs. What we believe can be very powerful in relation to how reality creates for us and how we live our experiences. A belief may begin in childhood or become instilled in us by others. As time goes on, it becomes buried further and further into our psyche. We begin to form behaviors around it, and ultimately, the belief can become a subconscious thing with a life of its own.

In fact, beliefs can be so strong that they are represented symbolically by a separate reality, such as an object or, in extreme cases, even as powerful creatures that act like guards to protect the secret of a belief within a client's energy field. As we believe, we feed energy to the belief. The strong reality of the belief begins to manifest as a separate form that lives in our Etheric field, parasitically living on our energy. The stronger the belief, the more alive it becomes. Beliefs can run the gamut of form from a static field of interfering energy to taking on an identity that represents the actual belief or a defense of the belief.

Thought Forms: The Monster in the Closet

Thought forms can affect an entire energy system, especially when the beliefs are not true. The hidden beliefs become sort of like the monster in the closet that many of us feared as a child. Only this time the monster is really there, hidden in the shadows of our very make-up. Thought forms first become alive as energy forms that manifest due to our strong beliefs. As those beliefs become ingrained within us, our thought forms literally begin to take on an other dimensional life of their own. When they are fear based, thought forms can take on some pretty ugly personalities. Thought forms can become animated as if they have taken on a life of their own. Some become so powerful they may even defend themselves. When that happens, thought forms can cause us all kinds of problems because they are sapping our energy, our life force. The key in these situations is to remember that thought forms are truly only symbols of beliefs, caricatures of true reality, and are only powerful to the one who holds the belief. Finding and eradicating a belief system in someone's energy field can change her life forever.

Fragmentation: Ethereally Falling Apart

Traumatic experiences in our history can cause us to fragment energetically. When we have a severe trauma or injury, certain parts of our energy system, particularly in the area of the throat and the solar plexus, can break into tiny pieces that look a lot like shattered glass. When that happens, our energy field is no longer cohesive, and we can become affected in various ways. We may become unable to focus for very long at a time, have a hard time making decisions, or experience large fluctuations in our emotional and physical energy levels. We might be happy one moment, depressed the next, or raring to go one minute, then suddenly need a nap.

When any part of our energy field has become fragmented, it looks much like broken glass. The energies start to break down and, in essence, break into

individual non-cohesive pieces that are no longer in correct form. Once fragmented, the area can no longer participate with the rest of the system. Instead,
the fragments become an aside, lost and disconnected.

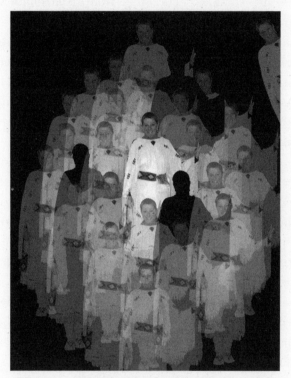

When our aspects become fragmented we lose full
cosmic communication.

Fragmentation can also happen on a soul level. A soul lives in multi-dimensional
levels of reality simultaneously. Usually, all of our multi-dimensional aspects work
together in a unified way that is a strong harmonic alignment of self. When parts of
the self become disharmonic, they move out of alignment.

Imagine a musical chord. Each individual part of that chord is a separate note,
an individual tone. When combined, those tones become a unified set of harmonics. If one of those tones is missing or is moved to a different position on the
scale, the result is that the chord does not sound complete or sounds disharmonic.
That is how our aspects work.

If each part of us is in alignment and in harmony, things go great for us. If part of us is closed off or out of alignment, our experiences are missing something or are not going well at all. When the soul fragments, any number of its individual multi-dimensional aspects can become disharmonic with the others and then misalign from the harmonics of the whole.

For example, a victim of child abuse may fragment during each event of abuse. The abuse is so traumatic that the child's aspects separate from each other in order to manage the intensity of the pain or emotions. The child learns to see himself as damaged, insignificant, or worse, so aspects of the child move out of alignment into a blocked off place so that the intensity of the pain does not have to be experienced.

Another example might be a teenager who feels so different and apart from his friends, that he completely alienates from himself and everyone during that time. When he does, his dimensional aspect that is that age sulks out of alignment or is closed off from the rest of the dimensional aspects and can remain forever caught in the negative feelings of that time.

He may eventually grow out of those feelings, but part of him has been walled off from the full pain of his experience. His soul is fragmented.

In less common cases, it is this kind of response to trauma that causes multiple personality disorder, or MPD. In its pain, the soul develops sectored aspects of itself that live separately one from the other.

Similarly, but in a much more acute sense, the same thing happens during post-traumatic stress. An experience happens in a split second that is so incomprehensible to the frame of reference of the person that his entire system literally explodes into thousands of tiny fragments. As the moment of trauma ends, the fragments spring back into place but remain not quite together in their original harmonic arrangement. The system begins to lack cohesion, is disconnected, and therefore, fragile. Any stimulus to the fragile system that is even a little bit similar to the original event then causes a similar reaction in the system. Until the fragmentation is assimilated, the system will react like a scratched record over and over again as it tries to correct itself by recreating its reaction over and over again.

Fragmentation can be pulled back together by an experienced multi-dimensional healer but only with the participation of the client. Some people call this soul retrieval. The soul really hasn't gone anywhere; it is just that its energy is fragmented. Instead, I call this assimilation.

Often there is a great deal of fear around post-traumatic stress and the feeling of being out of control is overwhelming. Post-traumatic stress disorder, or PTSD, is not about control at all, and that is why many methods of treatment have failed. In order to completely eradicate PTSD from an energy system, the fragments must be assimilated and re-harmonized.

Cloning and Transplants

There have been many attempts to clone living organisms, including animals. There are even possibilities discussed within the scientific world in relation to cloning people. Cloning is done by taking a sample of genetic tissue from a host organism and then growing a duplicate of the host based upon information in the host's DNA.

Cloning has been only partially successful because the cloned organism usually only lives for a short time and then dies of unexplained causes. The reason for this is that from a universal perspective, no two aspects of creation are or ever can be identical. Each individual set of tones, any form of manifested creation, is unique and holds a place in reality that is vital to the existence of reality.

By universal law, two identical aspects of creation cannot exist at the same time. One will cancel the other out, or they will both become so disharmonic that they cease to exist.

When a clone is created, it virtually carries the same harmonic frequencies and signature as its host. Because of that, the clone begins to subtly attempt to re-harmonize over time, but its genetic material attempts to maintain its original set of instructions. The clone is, in fact, destroying itself as it changes. The new harmonics are a bastardized form of truth and are disharmonic relative to creation. Ultimately, the newly cloned organism breaks down and perishes.

Remember how consciousness enters every embryo and later a fetus is formed? In the case of transplants, the organs of the host maintain some of the consciousness from the donor for a time. When the new organ is inserted into the recipient, the recipient may begin to have odd memories, emotions, or desires for certain foods, or sudden aversions to things they used to love. The consciousness of the host remains for an indefinite period of time but will eventually dissipate as cells are used up and more are generated from the recipient's body.

Trauma, Injuries, and Surgery

Our energy fields can become damaged in myriad ways, but often things that happen to us in our everyday lives contribute to the condition of our energy fields and our wellbeing or lack of it.

Trauma is something that we usually believe happens only emotionally or physically. For instance, an event happens in our life experience that we didn't see coming or that we don't have the life skills to deal with. Not only do we struggle emotionally, but our bodies also react chemically to protect themselves, and our energy fields move into different patterns in response.

Not only might our energy fields become rewired in their patterning as a reflexive defense, but some areas may become denser or even damaged, disconnected, or inflamed as a result of the trauma.

Further, when this happens, sometimes the trauma is so severe that our multidimensional aspects become fragmented. These different types of responses in our energy fields can happen on one level or many. It is often easy to read a person's field when there has been trauma because the trauma will land in specific areas of the field depending upon what kind it is.

From there, different stages of the Etheric anatomy are affected and, later, perhaps even dysfunctional. Indications of trauma can be found in the external field right from the beginning of a session. The external field, as we will learn later, is an elliptically shaped envelope of energy that holds us together. It is our first line of defense energetically.

When we are traumatized, our external field may become misshapen or bent in a specific area. In severe cases, it can even be torn. Then our energy field responds in different ways and begins to protect itself by fragmenting the trauma out to lessen its effects, becoming dense in some areas or even coming apart in extreme cases.

When we are physically injured, whether it is a minor injury or a severe accident such as a car crash, our energy field responds much in the same way as it does to trauma. The area of the injury becomes dense at the point of impact and may sometimes tear and begin to leak energy.

The consciousness has not yet registered the injury, so if it is gotten to immediately before the emotions come into play, that injury may be completely healed. Once the emotions become intertwined with the energy of the injury, the injury becomes a conscious part of the person and solidifies as a reality. In the form of a protective shell around the unwanted imperfection. When that happens, the injury or illness is difficult to heal.

The same thing is true of illnesses. Once the emotions become part of the mix, the illness is much harder to shake. Instead of the illness being seen as a part of the patient's experience, he sees it as a separate thing he must fight. If the entirety of the patient could first embrace the illness as part of his experience, he could change the experience by directing a new reality.

An extreme opposite example of these points is the case of someone who goes to the doctor, not feeling well but expecting a simple solution and a quick return to health. Once there, the doc tells him that he has a terminal disease and won't likely live for more than two weeks. Almost immediately, the patient begins to go downhill and on the fourteenth day, the patient dies because his emotions and beliefs have become part of his illness. Therefore, the illness must be the only experience possible, right? Not at all!

If the emotions and beliefs were changed, the reality would also follow suit.

In cases of surgery, different anomalies can develop in the external part of the Etheric field. The most obvious is that wherever an incision is made, damage is done to the energy field. The damage can run the gamut from a temporary indentation of the field to a full blown Etheric incision that will continue to leak energy. If, during surgery, a knowledgeable practitioner would be allowed to maintain balance of the energy field during the procedure, healing would be, not only more expedient, but often dramatically fast. Many hospitals are allowing their surgery staffs to run Reiki during surgery with good results. This is a fabulous development in the marriage of allopathic and alternative medicine! While it is a basic form of energy work, Reiki is a great start and does help to improve the patient's recovery and lessen the trauma from surgery.

Another problem that develops during surgery is the effect of the electromagnetic emissions of the surgical machinery and equipment in the room. Since the patient is anesthetized, she is, in effect, out of her body, changing the dynamics of how the energy field is reacting and responding to its environment. As a result of the electromagnetic energies in the room, the energy field may become interfered with or even rewired so that the energy patterns are in an unnatural flow pattern. In other instances, part or all of the Etheric field may become disharmonic and therefore remain in pain or sick, particularly in the area of the surgical procedure. The damaged area of the energy field can later develop into actual physical infection or irritation of the area.

While the patient is under anesthesia and unguarded by the force of her waking consciousness, she is also susceptible to picking up energies from everyone in the room. If a surgical tech, nurse, doctor, or other occupant is in a negative mood, feeling fragmented or tired, having an emotional day of any kind, the patient can literally pick up the same energy.

Further, the energy field often picks up electromagnetic anomalies from the environment that can create errors on the external wall of the patient's energy field. These look a lot like multi-armed stars of irregular shape and size. These energy attachments actually act as irritants to the external field and can literally cause physical pain and slow or incomplete healing.

The operating room for the patient is a very serious place as it is for some staff. For others it is just another day at the office where personal dynamics and moods abound. It would be a great idea for everyone to focus on the healing of the patient and to set the intentions and energy for the surgery from the outset so that the healing will be more efficient and complete.

Leaving the Body: Death Is Only a Transition

When we live in a human body, creation maintains our energy flow, filling us with consciousness and sharing from its infinite resources to keep us alive and healthy. In effect, we are drawing from our very source to live. There comes a time when we must leave our bodies, returning to the other side, no longer needing creation to sustain us as it had. When that moment comes, where do we go? What happens to all of that consciousness when we die? When our earthly bodies wear out and the time comes for our souls to move on? Again, I will tell you an amazing story:

One afternoon I received a somewhat desperate call from a friend and colleague of mine. She was traveling to be with her elderly father. The plan had been for her to pick him up and transport him to another state where he would reside in an assisted living facility and spend his last days near his family.

Before she arrived, my friend's 93-year-old dad slipped and fell and broke his neck. He had been rushed by ambulance to a hospital, where he was admitted to the intensive care ward and was failing fast. My friend called to see if there was anything that I could do to assist her dad in not only his comfort level, but in whatever was coming next. She felt as if her dad was going to die. She knew from our conversations that sometimes healing work isn't about fixing a problem but can also be about clearing the way so that a soul can make clear decisions to live or die with little to no effort.

I told my friend I would do what I could. Reading his energy through his daughter, I was easily able to tap into the dad's energy field. Accessing an unconscious or infirm person can be simple since their frequencies can be read through their connection with their loved ones. This concept may sound a bit complicated, but it is as easy as breathing once we become familiar with out of body consciousness.

I began to work with my friend's dad very gently, waiting for the energy field to reveal to me what was needed. I quickly discovered that this was one of those times when there wasn't anything I was supposed to fix, as this soul really was preparing to leave its body. I received the information that this session was about balancing the field and harmonizing its different layers to clear the way for this soul to do whatever was coming next.

I began to ethereally work, beginning with the area of the head. I gently worked my way through the Etheric system one step at a time. When I got to the level of the throat, an amazing thing happened. The chakra system, which is usually composed of a series of colored pyramids (more about this later), began to spontaneously change. Instead of glowing in their respective color harmonics, each was emitting a glow of golden light. I watched as a chain reaction went down the line from one chakra pyramid to the next. I was stunned. I had never seen an energy field act like this before. What was happening?

In the same instant that the question arose, it was answered. This man was in the early stages of dying. I sat back and exhaled one huge sigh. Wow. What a privilege to witness such a private moment in this soul's life. Wow.

Much in the same way that I had talked to the incoming soul, I asked this outgoing soul to show me what would happen throughout the process of his death.

He showed me that the rest of the chakras would convert to the golden energy and glow in unison with the others. Once this had occurred, harmonization throughout the complete system would be attained spontaneously. When full and complete harmonization was attained, an area of the external field would split open just above the heart area. As the opening progressed, the soul would release its grasp of the body, and wriggle out head first through the split in the external field. The soul would change dimensional realities.

Looking up through the split was similar to looking into the end of a tunnel with a light at the other end. The light was a field of energy where other souls awaited the arrival of their loved one. As the soul of the dying man moved closer to the light, he would be met and escorted by loved ones and other guides who would help him through his dying process.

What I witnessed was painless, easy, and joyous. There was no drama, no resistance—just a shedding of a dense body that no longer worked and a return into a light body form. The light that I saw was an aspect of our source light and it was filled with positive emotion.

This dear soul gave me an education that is beyond words. His daughter knew in her heart that her dad was leaving, and she only hoped to reach him in time to share his departure. She did, by the way, and he died less than two hours after I worked with him; having been brought back into full balance, he easily left his body to return to the light.

Later encounters with souls upon and after their crossing widened my understanding of the death process even further. I have learned that dying from the physical world is much like rising up from a deep scuba dive. The soul first leaves its physical body and then crosses over to the other side. It has merely shed its corporeal skin, the physical body. After that, it goes through various stages of debriefing, exploring the life it has just left and the people in it as well as the relationships, how the soul has affected others, and how they affected him.

There are life reviews, past life and future life reviews, periods of healing and harmonization, and an ultimate full return to the light. In each of the reviews, the soul is able to feel its effects on others. In each incidence of relationship that comes up in the life review, the soul feels the experience from the perspective of the others who were involved. This is a powerful and sometimes very profound or painful experience, as most often in life we never know how we have touched another.

During the time that the soul is transitioning from physical being back to light being, it may remain fully or partially aware of what is happening on earth. The departed can hear their loved ones and even contact them in various ways. The most common contact is in the dreams of their loved ones when they are relaxed and more available. Dreams of the departed are often actual contact from them.

Once the soul progresses past a certain point in its journey or returns fully to the light, however, it is no longer able to contact earthly reality, nor does it have a need to do so. Its journey is complete until the soul chooses to incarnate for another lifetime.

Death is a time when those of us who are left upon the earth feel great loss. The departed soul, on the other hand, at least in a normal, healthy crossing, soon learns that all of the little things in its earthly experience weren't that important in the overall picture and never really did matter.

What we need to realize is that in spite of generational teachings and common value systems, life isn't about achieving or a singular purpose or even a series of purposes. It is about living, pure and simple. When we live our lives fully, we are serving our purpose. We must embrace life in every moment and give ourselves the opportunity to experience every nuance it has to offer!

Soon after crossing, the soul returns to its most perfect image of self and, if it does appear to someone who remains on earth, may have the appearance of when the person was much younger, more vital, or healthier than when they were in their old age or sick or injured. For instance, when my dad passed away, he had been extremely sick for several years. He had had his leg amputated due to extreme diabetes and its effects, and his body had withered to a slight noth-ing. When he came to me at his funeral, he was young and vital looking, just like pictures I remembered seeing of him as a quarterback for Georgia Tech and, later, as an Air Force pilot. When my best friend Van passed away several years ago of acute leukemia, she came to me on her way out looking very much like her current age, smiling to tell me she was just fine. Later when she came to me in a dream, she looked about thirty years old, much like photos I had seen of her as a county commissioner, healthy and vital.

A soul who crosses over also soon forgets any negative emotions or challeng-ing relationships and carries with it a much wider and fuller perspective of the life the soul is leaving.

When one's essence is forced out of his body in instances of traumatic death, the transition may not be as smooth. Sometimes in the event of an accident or violent death, the soul may at first be confused, not realizing that its physical body has died. In these cases, the soul may remain on a plane close to our reality in a state of confusion as it tries to return home to its 3-D world. It may even be frustrated for a time, but ultimately the soul will generally realize what has happened and move on through its journey with actual relief.

Sometimes when a soul has been traumatically released from the body, it is left with a sense of life interrupted. In these cases, the soul will remain for a time until it feels that the unfinished issues have been resolved. The time that takes varies radically, depending upon the circumstances of each situation. Sometimes what keeps a soul from continuing on to the other side is a simple thing like words left unsaid, a task left undone, or emotions left unexpressed. Sometimes love is a great rein on the journey of a soul. The sheer passion of love and the departed's concerns for the remaining loved one can keep the departed soul earthbound. Other reasons can be much more complex and really not up to them at all. Once they realize this, the souls will go on their way.

There are many myths about suicide and what happens to the soul when someone takes his own life. Religions have varying stories of souls trapped on the inner planes forever or, worse, condemned for all eternity. None of this is true. I have worked with many families who have lost a loved one through suicide and have been able to talk with the departed loved ones about their intentions and experiences. Their remaining emotions are varied, but I was surprised to learn that the suicidal impulse was often spontaneous, an act of the moment, which reached a point of no return. It usually wasn't planned in advance, so there was nothing anyone could have noticed ahead of time or done to stop the suicide. Others had definitely planned their earthly release, but while the thought of suicide may occur, real planning is less common in my experience.

The important thing to know is that the souls of suicide victims (and yes, they are victims) cross over to the other side. Since they do not have a normal death process, the actual leaving of the body can be slower or, conversely, faster and not accomplished with as much ease, but the result is a crossing over nonetheless. Once the soul is free from its earthly life, it will go through many stages of realization and healing on the other side. Ultimately, the suicidal soul will return to its source just as all other souls do.

Grief can be a powerful deterrent to the afterlife journey of a soul. It can act as an energetic magnet pulling at a soul so strongly that it is literally held back from its journey to crossing over completely. We must realize that it is important to let our loved ones go. Believe it or not, we show them our love more by letting them go than we ever could have by holding them back.

Grief can also become so intensely powerful for the bereaved that it becomes resident within their energy fields, causing compression of energy, particularly in the abdominal area. The energy there becomes denser until the energy field becomes dysfunctional and the physical body becomes sick or diseased because the density restricts healthy energy flows.

Healing isn't always about a cure or a fix. Sometimes it is simply someone's time to leave. When someone is in the dying process, and healing is no longer an option for that soul, working with them ethereally can actually speed up the dying process. Once all the layers of the Etheric anatomy are aligned and the soul is getting a full flow of energy, and therefore instructions on all levels of communication, it is much easier for the soul to leave its body.

Working ethereally with someone as he is in the dying process does not kill him, but he may leave so quickly, either as you work or immediately after, that you might wonder. No, that is not the case. What you did by creating the necessary alignments and connections is to have cleared the way for that soul to choose clearly and easily to leave its body and go on to its next journey.

CHAPTER SEVEN

Energy and Exchanges

We now have a good idea of consciousness, energy, and creation, so it is time to begin to apply these concepts to real life. It is one thing to have an understanding but quite another to apply that understanding to life and healing.

How Energy Works

Energy is a living force of consciousness in action that is created by the movement of creation as it expends other energy.

We can think if it this way: When we move, we create a slight breeze. Creation is in a constant state of motion. It isn't going in a straight line; it is writhing, pulsing, and folding in upon itself all of the time. During all of that motion, energy is created, used, and re-created. It never stops.

All energy, as we learned earlier, moves in a spiral motion. As it was in the beginning and always is, energy comes in all frequencies and combinations of frequencies and seeks to join with other energy that is harmonically the same or similar. When those like energies connect, new reality is formed. As new reality is formed, it is reflected as different conditions of density depending upon the level of creation at which it occurs. No matter what level of reality a change occurs in, that change affects all other reality, and creation morphs to adjust to that new reality.

With each other and with everything around us, we constantly exchange energy. When we are with someone, we gain part of their energy, and they ours, and when we part, we are not the same as when we came together. We have been re-harmonized. Sometimes this feels wonderful and we feel up, happy, or even pleasant. Other times we feel very uncomfortable as if something isn't right in our world. When we feel good, it is because the other person was harmonically compatible with us. When we don't, the other person was not harmonic with us at all.

Exchanging Energy

One of the most important concepts that we can get out of all this information is that energy exchanges. In everything we do, with everyone we encounter or interact with, we exchange energy. We also exchange energy with our environment and with places. In each moment that we exist, we are never the same as we were the moment before because we are constantly harmonizing due to these exchanges.

A great real life example of how energy exchanges is when we are in a room full of people at a party. Everyone is having a terrific time, laughing, conversing, and becoming acquainted. A latecomer enters the room; she is stressed out and perhaps even angry at being delayed or at what caused the delay in the first place. Maybe she had a bad day, who knows?

As that person enters the room, she is emitting the energy of her emotions into the room and everyone there begins to feel her angst. Her anger. The intensity of her experience. Slowly, as the energy of her anger crosses the room, conversations begin to cease or slow down, people begin to stare, even hold their breath for a bit, and on the inside, those who were happy one minute and having a great time, all of a sudden feel less festive. That is because the intensity of the latecomer's energy field has actually entered into the energy fields of everyone else as it traveled through the room. A room that was functioning in harmony only a moment ago now becomes disharmonic.

When we encounter another person in any capacity, we exchange energy. The energy that each of us emits flows across the gap between us and enters our respective energy fields and flows between our respective particulates. This powerful event is extremely subtle but can affect us in mighty ways.

All of us have met someone who we instantly did not like or who caused us to be defensive or afraid for unknown reasons. That is because that person's energy was extremely disharmonic to us. Alternatively, when we meet someone for the first time and feel an instant bond, that person is harmonically compatible with us.

Not only do we experience those incoming and outbound energies in the moment of the experience, but some of the energy also remains residual within us for some time. When that happens, it either feels terrific and we feel happy and comfortable, or, conversely, we leave the encounter feeling inexplicably imbalanced or uncomfortable and perhaps even emotional although we can't explain what we are feeling or why.

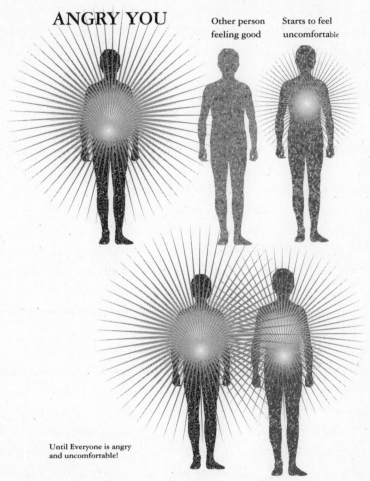

ANGRY YOU

Other person feeling good

Starts to feel uncomfortable

Until Everyone is angry and uncomfortable!

We convey everything not just in words but also energetically. When we are with other people, every single moment, we exchange energy. Whether we realize it or not we are greatly affected by the energy we receive from others and they by ours.

We also take in energy from others in a more direct way through an opening in our energy field called the solar plexus. Our solar plexus is located just below our diaphragm and serves many purposes; it is the entry point where energy from another person, place, or our environment enters into our system.

When that energy enters us, we are directly and immediately affected. When we are too open and leave our energy fields unprotected from the energy of others, we begin to inadvertently take on the energy of problems and issues that they are carrying. Usually this happens without our even realizing it. The exercise we learned to establish our Etheric protection, wherein we created a field of energy from our source light, can protect us from allowing unwanted energies to enter our energy fields.

In the same way that we exchange energy with other people, we also do it with our environment and places that we visit. No matter what we are doing, in every minute of our lives we are exchanging energy. There is no escape. We are part of a greater One, and within that membership our bodies and energy systems follow the same principles as all of creation.

I am often asked about life purpose. People have begun to seek their life purpose as if it is a one-time achievement in life.

Because of the way we exchange energy with everyone and everything, we are constantly in the flow of creation. We may never know how we have affected another person just in a brief passing, but we have, and they have changed us, and each of us will carry that change into our lives from that point on. The way we are affected may be a simple harmonization, or it could be a piece of information that the energy carried to or from us.

Because of the exchanges we share with all reality, we can see why it is important to be really present in any given moment. When we are, we become more aware of the subtle things that are happening within and around us, perhaps seeing signs that tell us how to make good choices or move in the direction we want to go in life. We may realize the need to be more intentional about our thoughts and actions and, in fact, any expression of energy that we make. Remember, that could be a word, an action, thought, virtually any expression of energy that we make as human beings.

Healing with Energy and Harmonics

When we use energy for healing, amazing things happen. Because it is a living form of consciousness, energy is intelligent and already knows where to go and what to do.

When we add an intention to that energy, the intention directs the energy specifically, based upon our intention. The energy gains purpose instead of being just a broad wave of energy that we sent without intention. Like a laser beam, intention directs energy to a specific goal or target.

When we add passion to an intention the passion acts as fuel to power the energy toward a directed cause.

Energy that is intentional and directed by passion is almost always perfectly effective . . . as long as the intention isn't so specific that it misdirects the energy to merge as a disharmonic error. If we have our own reasons for directing energy into the field of another, we can just about bet that whatever we are doing isn't going to work. Remember, energy knows what it is doing. It is a form of consciousness. When we instill that consciousness with an untruth, the energy will attempt to perform as we have directed it, but it won't work or, worse, will cause problems.

For example, say we have merged with the energy field of another person in the name of healing. Our energy, our consciousness, has combined with theirs for the moment. They have a pain in a certain area, and we have an opinion about why they have that pain or what is causing it. So we direct energy based purely upon our opinion. Not only does the pain not go away, it gets worse. Why? Because we have added more energy to the problem and inflamed it because our opinion was wrong to begin with!

When we are learning to use energy for healing and change, it is best to let the energy lead us.

Once we establish the flow of energy, if we have allowed ourselves to become sensitive to it and are aware of how the energy feels inside and around us, we can begin to recognize subtle changes that are occurring and direct our participation accordingly.

If allowed, our hands will flow like a symphony with the energy as it moves and seeks its destination.

Besides our opinions causing errors as energy flows, there are other things that can enhance or destroy even the best of intentions. Using external harmonics such as singing bowls or electronic frequencies can cause all kinds of disturbances in an energy field for either positive or negative, even devastating, results.

Right about now I know that many readers may be getting up in arms, but the truth is that external influences are also energy and affect everything in their sphere of influence. Sometimes they are so specific as a frequency or combination of frequencies that they can actually do harm, or they can effect a total cure. In our limited understanding of energy and its effects, we sometimes create energetic situations out of ignorance. In other cases, the product may not be perfectly tuned, so it is an error before it is even used.

For instance, assume that we have merged with the energy field of another, and we decide to use some form of frequency generator. We have been working all along and created a mutually beneficial energy space with our client. Because they are advertised to be effective or our friends have said good things about them, we decide to use, say, a specific tuning fork or bowl. We begin to play our new tool with all good intentions, but the singular frequencies that are emitted are totally wrong for that moment. The energy field of our client responds by closing up, changing the spaces between the particulates where all energy flows, and at the same time, traps that frequency in the system. That frequency is foreign to the system, so instead of helping our client, we have actually added an additional dysfunction!

The same goes for frequency generators, and there are many models on the market. They come with prepackaged frequency sets that can be directed into the client's energy field in various ways, either by sound, vibration, or light.

Most (not all) of these products are not beneficial to a human energy field, which is an intricate and infinite series of energy layers and grids that is harmonically attuned to all of creation. Its dysfunctions come from a variety of causes, and those dysfunctions are found in various areas and aspects of the person's harmonics. When a singular tone is introduced into such a fragile and finely tuned instrument that is us, it is like fingernails on a blackboard to our energy system. It can literally damage or even tear an area of the Etheric field.

Despite these things, a lot of positive good is being done with sound, vibration, and color therapies.

Like Dr. Rife's work in the 1930's, there are currently some terrific tools available, which if they are used correctly can truly enhance a healing process. Healing comes in all forms. It can be a simple awareness or a huge "aha." It can be a mental realization, an emotional process, a spiritual catharsis, or a physical progression, but it is never only one of these; it is always a combination of mental, emotional, spiritual, and physical aspects coming together harmonically toward perfection.

When delivering energy in any form (subtle energy flowing, sound, vibration, or even color frequencies) into someone's energy field, it is important to know never to deliver a singular frequency. All of these should only be delivered as harmonic sets. In other words, unless the tool is properly designed and creates harmonic overtones when used, never deliver a tone into anyone's reality!

So what to do instead? If you are truly guided, not mentally but intuitively, to utilize frequencies of any kind, use harmonic sets. In other words, more than one tuning fork at a time, or bowls that are perfectly tuned to create overtones when they are played. My friend, Beverly, at the Crystal Room in Mt. Shasta, California, makes the most incredibly accurate bowls I have ever experienced. Until the time I met her and experienced firsthand the perfect combinations of frequencies in the bowls she is manufacturing, I was completely against them. In fact, when first invited, I refused, telling her that I couldn't stand the disharmonies that bowls created in my energy field.

With a little coaxing from Bev, I went into her back room and was immediately transported into myriad realities and energetic experiences unlike anything I had ever experienced from external influences! The bowls are made of quartz combined with other precious and semi-precious minerals in various combinations. After they are fired, Bev tries them out, and if they are not perfectly tuned, she destroys them because she understands the effects of disharmonies.

Some of the bowls actually create multiple tones, and when the bowls are played in certain combinations, they create an effect of voices singing as if an Etheric choir were serenading us. One bowl that is a combination of quartz and three different minerals balanced all aspects of my being at once. It felt like a gentle Etheric snap as all of my energy instantly was attuned. Needless to say, I was in awe, and honestly had to reassess my opinions! While expensive, the purity of these bowls are a great positive toward our experience of color, sound, and vibrational healing.

Other great forms of energy healing are found in color therapy, music (definitely music!), and vibrations, such as drumming; in fact, there are unlimited ways that we can create energy for healing.

Using music in the healing space can have fantastic results on many levels depending upon the music that is chosen. It can not only help to relax our clients (and us), but music also communicates with our particulates and causes them to change their spacing. Music, when chosen properly, creates a widening between our particulates that allows the energies we introduce into our client's fields to move more rapidly, efficiently, and accurately to their destinations. Imagine. After all, music is living harmonics!

I am sure that there are other effective products to be found that can effect excellence in healing. Just be cautious in what you believe and use. Just because someone markets what I call gadgets with some magical uses doesn't mean they are for real or effective at all. Use discernment in all cases!

The same thing goes when we deliver energy through us to our clients. If we are following the energy, we will find that we are drawn to touch more than one place at a time. This is very important because when we do, we maintain harmonic balance in our client as we work.

When I first began touching bodies, my hands glided to specific areas. I began to see little lights on the bodies. They would usually be yellow (touch here!), red (inflamed energy that needed to be released) or shades of gray to black (energy stuck here). I never saw just one colored light. There were always multiples. I learned to touch them in the order that I saw them, and when I did, energy normalized, woke back up, or began to flow again. It was fascinating. Later I realized that I was working with harmonic sets and that when applied that way, they were extremely effective.

Each area that would light up may have been far from the previous one. I began to realize that I was working with the meridian lines and their subtle points. In the same way that acupuncture uses more than one needle, I was using my hands and fingers with the same results. I found that mentally understanding the harmonics was not only unnecessary, but impossible due to their subtleties; however, to follow what each body told me, unerringly brought positive and sometimes profound results.

The important fact to remember in any type of energy work is that *everything* is created of energy. That energy is created of light, color, sound, and vibration and is *specifically harmonic to the reality of each individual client*. No two are *ever* the same, *ever*. We may notice similarities in how the energy works or in our results, but each client is unique in all of creation and, therefore, *will require different energetic harmonics* than anyone else.

CHAPTER EIGHT

The Etheric Anatomy

NOTE This chapter, complete with color illustrations, can be found on the website for this book: www.redwheelweiser.com/p.php?id=50

Now that we have a good solid base of how consciousness works, how creation is formed, and how our consciousness works within that construct, we can begin to explore the Etheric anatomy.

The Etheric anatomy is composed of multiple fields and layers of energy. Each layer of energy in the Etheric anatomy contributes to the experience of the whole. If any area or level of energy is affected in any way, the overall experience can be changed.

The complexities of the overall field break down into easy to understand and read sub-parts. What these sub-parts have to tell us can actually give us an entire story about our client. In other words, every body and all its layers of reality tell a very clear and full story. When all put together, the details of that story can be amazing in their accuracy.

In order to fully portray the systems, we will go through each area of the Etheric anatomy separately, slowly building a full and complete picture of the complexities that compose how we are made.

The External Field

When we first access another person, we encounter the external field. This area basically establishes our "personal space." When people stand too close to us, they are literally standing in our energy field, and that is not usually very comfortable for us. This field is an elliptical body of energy that envelops us much like a cocoon. The external field is our connection to creation in every respect. It acts as a translation station for both incoming and outgoing energy and information.

The information that comes to us via all of the tiny hallways in creation, filters into our external field and ultimately into us. As the information processes though the outer walls of our external fields, it becomes harmonized so that our systems can recognize and interpret it. Information about our past, present, and future and everything that is happening within creation is coming into our Etheric systems all of the time. Further, information about all of creation and what is happening within it is coming into us. At the same time, information about our life experience constantly flows back outward into the creative process, informing the rest of creation about our journeys. Every bit of the information flows in the form of energy.

Our external fields, when healthy, are filled with combinations of harmonic frequencies (different tones of energy) that flow in a very liquid manner.

NOTE The illustrations that accompany this chapter can be viewed in color on the website for this book, http://www.redwheelweiser.com/p.php?id=50

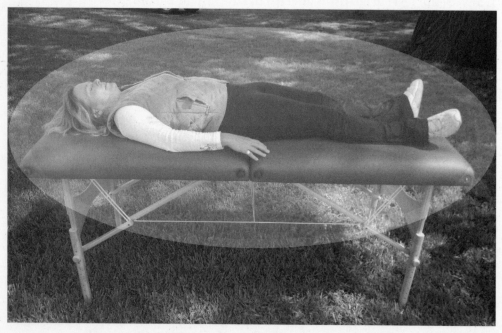

The external field has two layers and surrounds us like a cocoon.

Our external fields have an interior envelope, a smaller version of the most outer field, with what I call a soft wall around it. The chakras are connected to the interior, softer wall. Energy that is distributed from the chakras flows outward, first into the outermost part of the external field, and then through its wall into creation.

The external wall reflects light. The light that is reflected is what we often call *aura*. Many people mistake the aura for the external field, but this is not true. Intuitives who are able to see auras are seeing light as it reflects off the outer wall of the external field. The internal condition of what is contained within that field, in conjunction with external stimulus to our systems, reflects light of changing colors, depending on what is happening in our field at any given moment. When a person is feeling very intense, or even angry, or perhaps extremely expressive, the aura will reflect red energy.

In times of great mental exercise, overthinking, or mental inspiration, the field will reflect bright yellow color. Love is generally very rosy pink, while someone who is highly spiritual will reflect violet or white energies. Healing energies can be blue or green, while orange is very expressive, and purple creative. There are many variances to these colors and how they combine to create a full-blown aura.

The external field also has specific positions on its outer wall that I call *axiom points*. These points are intermittent and evenly spaced all around the outside wall of the external field.

The axiom points are very important as they are our connection to the universal grid lines of energy flow, which are an infinitely reaching system of overlapping avenues of energy that, in a way, are a great pipeline of energy and information throughout all of creation. The grid lines ultimately refine, becoming smaller and smaller and more intricately woven until they connect within our personal energy systems to feed our meridian systems, which are small but very vital pathways of energy within our bodies.

When we are working on the exterior field, all we need to do to shift the whole field is to find the axiom points along the exterior of the field. If we tune these up, the whole field can become balanced.

The outer wall of our external energy field can become damaged for different reasons. When we suffer a traumatic injury or severe physical trauma, this part of our Etheric anatomy may actually become dented or torn, or the entire external envelope may become misshapen. When this occurs, the dented area becomes very dense, and the energy on the inside of the field does not flow in its normal directions or with its normal fluid motion. Instead, the energy will begin to reroute and ultimately small individual offshoots of energy may occur. I have seen the interior of the external field become completely filled with little errant spirals of energy that don't go anywhere.

When the external field becomes torn, vital energy leaks out slowly and the person will feel lethargic, have trouble healing or maintaining a decent energy level in everyday life.

Belief systems show up in this field in different ways, sometimes as dense blockages or symbols that have taken form or even animated in order to represent the belief and the emotions behind them. Belief systems can also cause matrixing, or entanglement of the internal energies, and interrupt flow within this field.

Our external energy field also tends to collect Etheric junk, formations of energy that do not belong to the person at all. Some cultures call this nebulous trash dross. This kind of energy is foreign to the field. It has no use and no

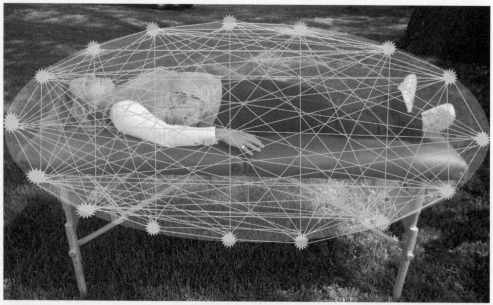

The external field with axiom points around the exterior that connects our personal grid system with the grid system of creation.

apparent reason or origin and can become caught in the field like sandspurs, irritating the field in general and creating inflammation. Depending upon the area where it is found, the location of this cosmic junk may manifest as pain or discomfort in the physical body respective to its position.

The Pranic Tube

Our pranic tube is our widest channel, or pipeline of energy. It is our greatest internal energy highway. The pranic tube is connected to both the top and bottom of our external field by vortexes of energy that flow into the pranic tube.

The energy that flows into the top of our pranic tube is cosmic energy, the energy of creation and all that it contains. This energy is very high frequency and feels very light. The energy that flows up into the tube from below is earth energy, a force of energy that maintains our balance with the earth. Earth energy is much heavier than the cosmic energy and in comparison feels a lot like molasses.

These two powerful energies meet in the middle of the body at the level of the solar plexus and are then mixed and distributed through the chakra and meridian systems. A constant flow of mixed energy is fed through the chakras. As the chakras distribute the energy, it is further distributed into the meridian system

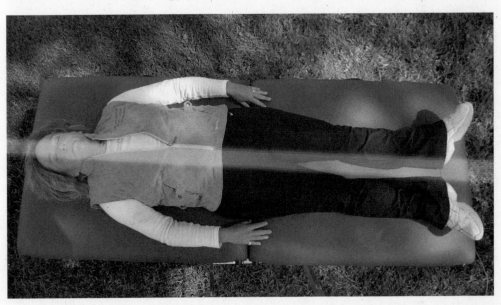

where the energy is carried throughout the physical body, feeding and nourishing it. The combination of the cosmic and earth energies creates the essence of the life force of human energy.

The flow of energy into the pranic tube is constant unless for some reason the vortex where the energy enters becomes damaged, bent, or inverted. Believe it or not, this happens quite commonly but is easy to repair.

The Truth about the Chakra System: It Is a Big Deal!

The chakra system has been mistaken as a series of rotating disks of energy that reside in certain areas of the body. Being able to see energy in the way that I do, I soon realized that the chakras, when healthy, are actually shaped like four-sided pyramids. Each is a different color, depending upon its position on the body. Contrary to popular belief, the chakras of both males and females rotate in a clockwise manner. They are not only on the front of our bodies, we have them in the back too.

Within each chakra pyramid is a vortex of energy that normally rotates clockwise, drawing energy up from the pranic tube and distributing it around the chakra's respective area of the body and also into the external field. It is this clockwise motion that has often been mistaken as a revolving disk.

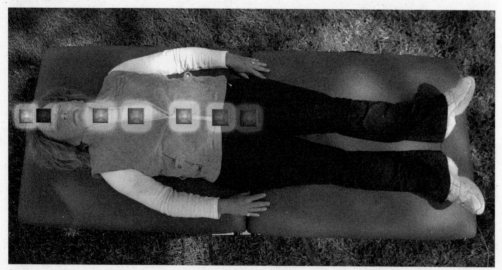

Chakra alignment top view.

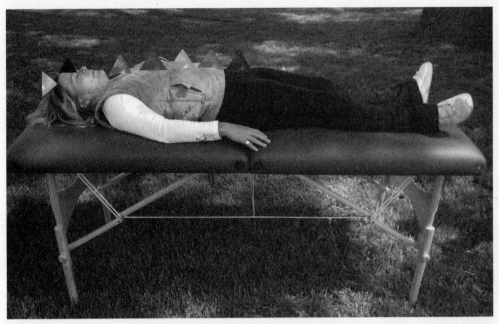

Chakra alignment side view of pyramids.

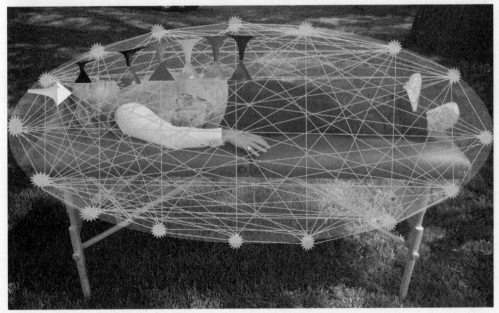

Chakras connect to the interior wall of the external field.

Chakras also have apertures much like a camera or a blinking eye. The apertures modulate energy flow as it moves through that particular chakra area. Sometimes the apertures can become stuck in a particular position. When that happens, energy may be restricted, cut off, or conversely, flowing too much.

Each chakra has immense purpose relative to our life experience and is also related to different parts of our physical body. We will address the main seven chakras. There are actually more chakras, which have to do with finer aspects of our Etheric anatomy, but I have found that when I completely address the seven most basic chakras, the more Etheric ones spontaneously harmonize on their own.

For example, a chakra may become reversed in polarity, changing its rotation pattern from clockwise to a counter-clockwise flow. When this occurs energy is actually being drawn from the overall system like a drain in a bathtub.

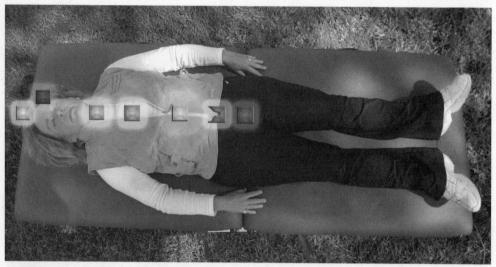

Chakras may become damaged in many ways. They may also become dysfunctional for many reasons. Some problems affect only specific chakras while other problems can affect all or several of them. Chakra anomalies: Note that the third eye chakra is off center, above its normal plane and out of alignment with the rest of the chakra system. The solar plexus is very inflamed, and the second chakra is torn. These are common anomalies in the chakra system.

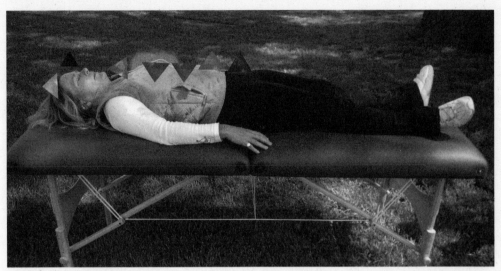

Chakras can malfunction in a variety of ways. Notice how the crown chakra has reversed and changed color. This anomaly is often seen in very mental people. The third eye pyramid has lifted away from the body and disconnected. This happened because the crown chakra was malfunctioning. Note the throat chakra has tilted, or angulated away from its base. The heart chakra has flipped and is sunken down into the body. Its energy is mostly on the surface. The heart chakra is now acting as a drain on the energy field and this person is likely living on the surface, not letting people see her inner self. The solar plexus, which is usually yellow, has sunken down into the body as a self-defensive measure and is blocked.

When someone is feeling self-defensive about a certain issue, the chakra that is related to that issue or a combination of chakras may sink too deeply into the body. When this happens, the energy of that area of the body becomes low in both amount and functioning and other problems may begin to occur.

A chakra may also become angulated, leaning out of position. When it is, the energy force becomes out of alignment, and errors of direction of the flow in energy will occur.

The chakras actually create an electromagnetic field of energy that maintains the spacing and positions of the meridians, or smaller pathways throughout the body. These pathways may actually move closer and closer to the center of the body during a time of low chakra energy and begin to stick together. I call this matrixing. It looks a lot like a star of energy lines that are uneven and going in a lot of different directions. When the meridian lines matrix by becoming stuck together, the normal pathways of energy are interrupted and energy is send in errant directions.

The vortex within a chakra might become fragmented, particularly in the areas of the throat and solar plexus. I will discuss this more when describing the function of each chakra individually.

A chakra may begin to bleed energy, becoming disorganized of form and covering the surface of the area of its position. A chakra may also become blocked or inflamed until its energy flow becomes still, then stagnant, or expanded to an uncomfortable inflamed state.

The vortex inside of a chakra may also become too long or too short and the chakra then rotates out of balance. A chakra vortex that has extended and elongated usually means that the person is looking outside of themselves for validation about specific kinds of things. As they reach their energy outward, the energy of the related chakra becomes stretched and remains elongated.

One that is too short can be caused by problems in surrounding areas of the Etheric anatomy. When a chakra is shortened, it becomes too dense and its rotation is slowed way down. Either way recalibrating the vortex to normal size is also easy to do.

Chakras may also become disharmonic, no longer in tune with the rest of the body. When this occurs, the chakras actually become the wrong color and sometimes even exhibit combinations of color when a chakra attempts to normalize its error. Changing the harmonic frequency of a chakra pyramid is called attunement. In a way, attuning a chakra is a lot like tuning the strings of a musical instrument. We do this by intention.

The interior of a chakra vortex may also become clogged with debris that the system has picked up externally as well as by energies that have crystallized. This can occur for a variety of reasons. Crystallized energies look a lot like tiny little bars of energy that reflect different colors. They are much harder in density than the chakras and can act as irritants within the chakra. Irritation that is caused by crystallized energy can actually affect the physical body and its organs.

Sometimes in extreme cases, a chakra might shut down completely. When that happens, there are almost always physical symptoms that accompany the chakra dysfunction.

Certain chakras, particularly the second one, may become torn into one or more sections. This is a severe anomaly since, when it is torn, a chakra essentially loses all of its energy.

All chakras can be affected by electromagnetic energy in the environment. When we spend time in places where there is a lot of excess electromagnetic energy, such as offices and hospitals, different areas of the energy field will become contaminated and begin to show different types of anomalies, such as thickening or matrixing on the outer walls of the external field or misplacement of chakra vortexes.

Power lines are another powerful source of electromagnetic interference; as the electricity runs through the wires, electromagnetic energy is thrown off from the lines. This can happen to varying degrees and affects all living things in the area.

I have also seen different affectations in the energy fields of people who have had surgery. Certain events occur during surgery that leave our energy fields unprotected, as well as exposed to electromagnetic pollution.

Chakras have three basic types of alignment. The first alignment is to the center. The centerline follows the exact center of the body so that the chakra can link with the pranic tube.

The second is alignment to plane. The chakra should sit just a hair below skin level. When it becomes too deep, this is an indication of self-defensive posturing. We will most likely find later correlation to the causal issue in a different location of the energy field.

When a chakra rises up off of its rooted position, it often will also float off to one side or the other of the centerline. This can be caused by a number of things including imbalance in that area of a person's life, a strong belief, electromagnetic pollution in one's environment, or even a physical injury. Chakras are, when normal, firmly rooted in place, with a good seal around the base to prevent energy leakage.

The third kind of alignment is the angulation of the pyramid. The pyramid and its vortex, when normally placed, will sit straight up at a 90-degree angle to the centerline. The pyramid may become angulated for any number of reasons, and when it is, the energy flow is slowed or interrupted. If the pyramid becomes angulated too far, the energy inside of the pyramid begins to leak out around the bottom of the uprooted pyramid.

Any area of the body, including the chakras, may have more than one dysfunction going on at any time. In order to effect the greatest change, it is best to work with the outermost affectation first and then work deeper for each repair. This is a lot like peeling an onion. Sometimes outer affectations cloud or block access to deeper dysfunctions. And once we take care of the outer layer, a new dysfunction is revealed that we can then address.

To best explain the chakras and their most common dysfunctions, let's explore each one individually.

The Crown Chakra

The healthy color is white. It is harmonic with the throat, solar plexus, and root chakras. This chakra is relative to the brain, the upper sinuses, and the pituitary, pineal, and hypothalamus glands. It is the vortex entry point for incoming cosmic energy to the pranic tube. The incoming energy carries information. It also cleanses and refreshes the system so that the body and surrounding energy systems remain fully functional.

The crown chakra is most affected by overuse of mental faculties. As we use all that electrical energy in our brains, its intensity causes dysfunction of the more subtle energies. When mental use becomes out of balance, the energy within the entire crown chakra becomes very yellow, the color of mental energy.

This vortex may also become inverted, or upside down. When this happens, the vortex is no longer receiving fresh energy and instead, blocks the flow of incoming energies.

The crown chakra may also become bent to varying degrees or angulated out of position.

It may also elongate in cases where the client does not trust her ideas and opinions and constantly seeks the opinions of others.

The Third Eye Chakra

The color varies from shades of indigo blue to a blue violet, depending upon the person. The third eye vortex is relative to the eyes, ears, and lower sinuses. It is immediately affected if the crown chakra is dysfunctional.

The third eye chakra is harmonic with the heart and the second chakra. This vortex is a portal to higher consciousness.

The third eye vortex is most affected by our beliefs and resistances about accessing other worlds. If a gifted child is told that the gifts aren't real or becomes frightened and then shuts the gifts down, a nebulous blockage forms and floats just above the apex of the pyramid, blocking the sight. This is kind of like static that interferes with a radio signal so the signal becomes unclear or interrupted.

If the crown vortex is out of balance in any way, the third eye will almost always be affected. This vortex may move off center and may very often be found floating above its normal placement, usually but not always to the left side of center.

On a few rare occasions, I have seen this vortex invert and become reversed in polarity. Usually if this has happens, the crown vortex is very affected in some way as well.

The Throat Vortex

The color is icy blue. This chakra is relative to the voice, throat, shoulders, neck, and extreme upper back. The throat vortex is relative to issues of trust, control, trauma, and feeling safe to speak one's inner truth. It is also relative to our multi-dimensional aspects and an indicator whether those aspects are in alignment or not. This vortex is harmonic with the solar plexus and root chakras.

The throat vortex is also in an area where several of the meridian lines pass closely together. This exquisitely harmonized area is one of the most likely to become dysfunctional.

The throat chakra is usually the first to fragment, often in response to trauma or when the client has deep-seated feelings of personal insignificance or is lacking personal power. The fragmentation in this area is also a sign that there is fragmentation, or a misalignment, of one's multi-dimensional aspects.

The throat vortex may invert, becoming of reverse polarity, flowing counter-clockwise. When this happens, energy is draining out of the system.

This vortex may also misalign off center or plane and can angulate to any degree.

The throat is the first vortex area that may matrix. When it becomes weak from any issue, the lowered expression of energy from the vortex no longer holds the meridian lines in place. They start to move out of position, falling toward the center, seeking energy. The meridian lines ultimately land in the center, above the pranic tube. Since there is nothing holding them in place, the meridian lines may become entangled or stuck together as they attempt to gather energy for the body anywhere they can. Entangled, the meridian lines begin sending energy in every direction except the correct one.

The Heart Chakra

The color is very bright leprechaun green. It is harmonic with the third eye and second chakras. The energy of this pyramid relates to the heart and lungs, breasts and mid-back. It is relative to the emotions and one's emotional self-defenses.

The heart chakra is quick to bleed energy in cases of unresolved emotions. When it does, the energy usually looks like pools of green on the surface. This affectation indicates that the client is living life on the surface, not allowing relationships on a deeper level that expose his true feelings. He lives from a state of reserved or hidden emotion because somehow he feels that it is safer than revealing his deeper, more private, emotions. When I see this, I usually tell the client that what doesn't get in also doesn't get out and that life emotions don't need to be edited, but felt and experienced to their fullest.

The heart chakra may become withdrawn into the body as a self-defensive posturing, and when this happens, it may remain upright or become inverted and of reverse polarity. When the heart chakra becomes inverted, it is a major drain on the energy system. Usually when a vortex is inverted, there will also be blockage inside the vortex, as if it is plugged. When there are vortex blockages, there may also be blockages of varying thicknesses literally over the vortex opening or in the surrounding area. For example, if the heart vortex is blocked, the chances are good that the chest area will display blockages in the areas around the vortex location. The area beneath the vortex may also become blocked. If the heart chakra is blocked, it is always wise to check the rest of the chest area, as there will almost always be other significant blockage there too.

The Solar Plexus

The color is a deep rich yellow. This vortex is relative to most of the internal organs, including the stomach, small intestine, diaphragm, gallbladder, liver, and spleen. It is relative to issues of relationship, creativity, and self-expression. This chakra is perhaps the most important of all as it has multiple functions and can be greatly affected with different anomalies. It is most harmonic with the throat. Often anomalies found in the solar plexus have already demonstrated in the throat.

Not only is this chakra relative to certain organs and issues, it is the area of the body where the down flowing cosmic energy and the up flowing earth energies meet and are mixed and distributed. This is a vital point in the overall energy system because if it becomes damaged or dysfunctional, the distribution of powerful energies through the body becomes crippled or inhibited, and the entire system is affected.

The solar plexus is also the area of the body where energy from other people, the environment, and events enter the system. It is like an aperture, a portal, a doorway to the entire energy system. This chakra tends to have multiple anomalies when dysfunctional and must be worked from the outermost to the innermost, one layer of dysfunction at a time.

The solar plexus area, or mid-section of the body, is also where unexpressed anger in the form of inflamed, red, and often hot energy is stored. When anger is withheld in any situation and not expressed or dealt with, it becomes filed away within the body. This can later cause real problems, particularly in the liver, upper digestive tract, gallbladder, and stomach.

Unexpressed emotion, especially grief, may also be stored in this part of the body. When we do not allow ourselves to move through our grief or to process our emotions, when we don't have the tools to deal with life's crises, when we experience uncomfortable or traumatic emotions, we tend to hold our breath, become tense, and as we do we clamp down on ourselves, compressing our energies. When we do this, the energy of the emotion becomes trapped, lodged in our energy fields, and then over time becomes compacted and dense.

The solar plexus chakra may become inverted, acting as a drain on the system. The interior of this vortex often becomes clogged with debris in the form of crystallized energies that look like tiny splinters and actually irritate the interior of the vortex, sticking like thorns into the inside walls of the vortex.

Angulation of the solar plexus vortex is common and requires correction.

The solar plexus can become deeply blocked. As we defend ourselves emotionally or experience fear, the solar plexus portal closes momentarily, blocking energy flow. When that occurs, the internal energy of the pyramid may become compacted and dense, inhibiting the energy flow.

Similar to the heart vortex, the solar plexus generally is blocked somewhere outside of the actual chakra position, in the upper abdominal area. Blockages in the surrounding solar plexus areas are generally moderate to severe and may be located just on the surface or positioned downward, deep in the body.

Fragmentation is common in this area. If there is fragmentation of the solar plexus chakra, you can just about guarantee there is also fragmentation in the throat area. When the chakra becomes fragmented, it is like broken glass. With no container to hold it, the energy leaks out in multiple directions and the vortex becomes broken into individualized pieces rather than being unified, cohesive, and functional.

The solar plexus vortex is quick to invert and become reversed in polarity when issues arise that we won't or cannot deal with. The vortex may even sink way into the body and be difficult to find. When it does, the meridian lines matrix all across the opening of the upside down vortex, further sending energy in errant directions. When the vortex sinks like this, it is a self-defensive posturing, and the client is usually very damaged in issues of relationship, creativity, or self-expression and unable to communicate feelings or perceptions easily. Instead, the client feels unsafe even in general types of relationships. She may even tend to isolate and be anti-social.

Occasionally when accessing the solar plexus, we may receive information regarding past lives of the client. When this happens, the previous life is usually relevant to the issues the client is experiencing in the current life. When revealed, the past life information is very specific about an event or emotion that was unresolved and continues to challenge the client even in his current lifetime.

The Second Chakra

The color is a warm, medium orange. This chakra is relative to issues of how one sees oneself and how one believes others see her. This chakra affects the reproductive organs, kidneys, bladder, and most of the large intestine. Contrary to most of the chakra charts, I find that this chakra also indicates sexual issues and is most often where issues of both sexual and emotional abuse are revealed.

The second chakra is easily affected by self-doubt and situations of conflict as well as issues of lack, feelings of invalidation, and loss of self-worth. Anomalies to the second chakra vary widely, although this chakra never matrixes.

Fragmentation can occur, but more often than fragmenting, this chakra will literally tear into two or three sections that remain attached to the base. When this occurs, it looks a lot like a torn kite that has been ripped by the wind. In cases of extensive tearing, one should suspect trauma that may involve sexual, mental, or emotional abuse, sometimes all three. At the very least, a severe trauma or series of traumas has occurred that affect that person's feelings of self-worth.

The second chakra can fall out of alignment easily and will also be drawn into the body. It may become weak in charge, looking diluted and a much lighter shade of orange to the point that it becomes transparent. If the solar plexus is affected, this chakra is nearly always dysfunctional in some way.

Angulation is often found in the second chakra too, as well as blockages of varying degrees. Withheld emotion may even be found this low if there is a severe amount in the solar plexus. Grief will often store in the area in addition to or instead of in the solar plexus area. The second chakra is harmonic with the heart, so when self-defensive indications are found there, they will likely be found in the second chakra as well.

The First Chakra

Color is bright red but may be very dark red when energy flow is interrupted in the chakras above. This chakra is relative to sexual function and sex organs as well as the anus. This area is relative to one's feelings of belonging, fitting in, and issues of general as well as physical safety.

The first chakra often becomes very dark when there is dysfunction either above it or of this chakra. It will sink partway into the body or become misaligned. I have never seen a first chakra fragment or matrix. The first chakra may angulate out of position, but if it does, it usually remains at least partially rooted.

Kundalini

Kundalini is a double helix of energy. It is a two-strand force that is a continuous flow of energy. The kundalini helix looks a lot like a DNA strand, or a chain. It begins at the root chakra, or base of the spine, and moves in a serpentine motion around the chakras.

The kundalini picks up energy from each of the chakras and carries it up and down through the body in a never-ending flow. This process helps keep the energy flow throughout the body in balance. When we reach certain higher states of consciousness, the kundalini energy rises higher and higher in our bodies and can ultimately unify all of the areas of the chakra system in an integrated and expanded force of energy. In a way, the kundalini is the Gamma Consciousness

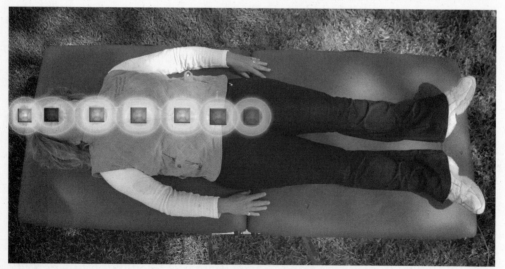

Kundalini is a chain of endlessly flowing energy through the center of our body. The width of expression of Kundalini is exaggerated in this photo. As it snakes its way up the body, the serpentine movement of each of the two kundalini strands wind their ways around each of the chakras.

of the body. As we access higher levels of Gamma Consciousness, our kundalini responds just as our DNA does. It begins to rotate faster, rising higher, extending its spiral from our root at the end of our spine up and out through the crown of our head.

When the kundalini is expanded in this way, amazing things happen to our senses and our bodies. The third eye aperture can open fully, as does our crown vortex, and we can experience the world as if looking from above our heads rather than through our physical eyes.

When the kundalini is accessed and expanded, sexual energy runs very intensely, and spontaneous orgasms can occur. The more a person works with energy and opens the flow of kundalini through his body, the more active the kundalini becomes. This can feel like an incredibly intense sexual experience, but a word of caution here. This is not the same as physical sexual stimulation even though sex can be enhanced by expanded and risen kundalini; it is a fully encompassing physical, spiritual, and energetic experience. With some practice, one can learn to control this force to enhance both intuitive and sexual experiences.

When we experience kundalini rising, it is easy to become confused about the intensity of sexual stimulation that spontaneously occurs. Often when I teach classes about ethereal healing and consciousness, I get a phone call within a few weeks from embarrassed student who shyly reveal to me that they are having a large degree of sexual stimulation when using the healing process. Kundalini energy can feel extremely sexual but must not be mistaken for sexual desire for another person. Kundalini sexuality is very personal. It should not be interpreted as something that has to involve another person for release. On the contrary, kundalini energy can be combined intentionally on our own or with another consenting adult for amazingly heightened sexual experiences. This is called Tantric sex and can be enhanced by using different techniques and positions as well as expressions of different energy frequencies.

When there are dysfunctions in the energy system, such as a malfunctioning chakra, the kundalini energy stays low in the body, and we feel very grounded. As we reach into higher levels of consciousness, our energy fields respond and our kundalini then rises unobstructed.

If there are dense blockages, leakages, or other anomalies in our energy systems, the kundalini chain may actually become broken. When this happens, the entire energy system becomes skewed in its flow, and the energy pathways move to compensate for the errors. Whenever the energy pathways move to adjust the energy flow, some part of our system isn't getting cleansed, balanced, and fed so that it is healthy. Ultimately we can become physically ill.

I have often seen the kundalini fall into a crumpled heap at the bottom of the body. This occurs when several of the chakras are dysfunctional. Lowered kundalini creates problems in awareness as well as inter-body communication. It can also generate a low libido and low functioning of different parts within the body.

The kundalini chain can be repaired in the same way other parts of our energy system can. When a practitioner is not accustomed to tapping into the energy flow of the kundalini, it may actually make him dizzy or cause a momentary loss of balance. Once acclimated to the kundalini flow of the client, however, the practitioner can follow the chain with his consciousness, looking for errors or breaks in the chain. Once found, the problems can be corrected by commanding that the chain normalize, assimilate (to reattach broken aspects of the chain) or rise (when it has fallen to the bottom of the body).

The Etheric Bodies

The Etheric bodies are quite beautiful and, depending upon their positions, are of different colors and functions. Except for the higher, causal bodies, the Etheric bodies stack in a particular order directly above and aligned with the physical body.

The Etheric bodies are sometimes carried in a nested manner and, if left that way, are difficult to read. It is easy to raise them by spreading our hands palms up over the physical body and asking them to rise up. As we then slowly raise our hands upward, the Etheric bodies will separate from each other and levitate above the physical body in a specific order.

Since we are immersed in the client's energy field, the Etheric bodies easily respond. In the moment that the bodies arise in this manner, the client, if relaxed, will literally leap out of her body temporarily.

One way to tell that someone has leapt out is that they will begin to snore very softly and their breathing will become very slow and shallow. It is vital to watch the client carefully while we work because sometimes when someone's body is so relaxed and they are traveling outside of it, they may stop breathing momentarily.

Being out of body is a blissful state, which may not be remembered, but some-times the client is so relieved to be out of a painful body, and it feels so good, it can be difficult for them to want to come back. It is extremely important not to startle the client during this time. Keeping a hand on the client at all times helps them maintain a connection to their body. If it becomes necessary to call them back to their body when we are finished working, a light touch accompanied by a soft voice will usually do it. Usually, I touch the client's arm or shoulder, lean over quietly, and ask if anyone is home. The client may not be able to respond at first, and if they don't, there is no need to panic. Wait a minute or two to give them a chance to become more aware again. Then ask them again to come on back. Sometimes it takes a few times, but they will reenter their bodies.

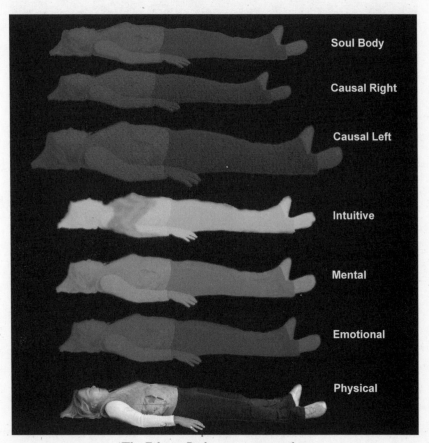

The Etheric Bodies in correct order.

The first sign that the client is reentering her body comes with a tiny movement of the toes or the tips of the fingers. Then the feet flex at the ankles and the person begins to flex her fingers. The client may not be able to move until she is more firmly seated in her body. Care must be taken when she sits up because she may be disoriented for a few minutes. This is because she is in a new state of balance and her center may feel different.

This experience is amazing for clients, but they tend to be very spacey for a while afterward, so I usually sit people down and give them a glass of water until they are totally oriented. This feeling is a high unlike any drug can offer, and

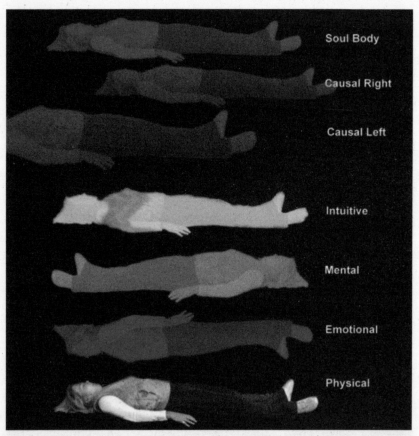

Misalignments of the Etheric bodies. Note that the emotional body has flipped over, the mental body has reversed position and the causal bodies are out of alignment on parallel.

driving in this condition can be unsafe, so we really need to make certain our clients are safe before they leave us.

The Etheric bodies have three types of alignment: center, plane, and parallel. A healthy well-aligned Etheric body will be aligned at exactly the center of the physical body, lie level on its appropriate plane, with the head and feet exactly in the same position in alignment as the physical body. Occasionally, a system has harmonized in a way that one or more Etheric bodies are reversed, with the head in the feet position. If so, this is usually normal for that particular system's harmonic arrangement, and we don't need to change the position of the body or bodies.

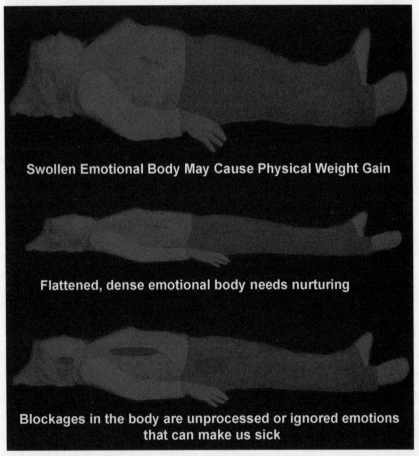

Errors specific to the emotional body can cause physical symptoms and even disease.

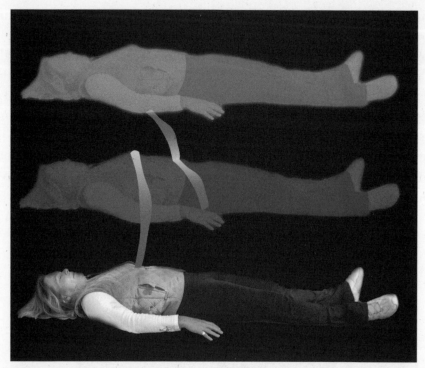

Sometimes as a self-defense mechanism, the physical, emotional, and mental bodies may become corded together. When this happens, our emotions and our mental perceptions become mixed up and we lose clarity. The energies become entangled as well, and we lose much of our cosmic connection as well as our sensitivities.

The Etheric bodies serve many purposes, specific to each respective body. What is found in, on, or around the Etheric bodies can correlate with information that is found in the chakra system. The two closest bodies, the emotional and the mental, are usually the most greatly affected. They show dysfunction more quickly and are most likely to have a direct effect on the physical body.

The farther out in alignment a body is, the higher dimensional it is. Events in the third-dimensional world usually affect the mental and emotional bodies, and don't go beyond them. Conversely, the farther out the body is, the older or more soul-oriented the affectation. I will explain more fully as we discuss each body.

The Etheric bodies can be accessed and scanned with the hands in the same way the physical body can be scanned. You might feel warm and cold spots in these bodies in the same way that they are felt on the physical body. We will talk about this more in depth in a little while.

Like our physical bodies, each Etheric body has its own set of otherworldly bodies. I have found, though, that if we work with the immediately related Etheric bodies, the secondary bodies will attune spontaneously, so there is no need to be concerned about those at this time.

It is common to find anomalies in the Etheric bodies that directly contribute to acute or chronic situations in the physical body as well as the life experience. Anomalies in the Etheric bodies can actually cause chaos in life, difficulty in manifesting or creating change, repetitive experiences, and general dissatisfaction. When the anomalies are repaired or cleared from these bodies, life changes almost immediately, and the client begins to see greatly positive trends and changes.

The Emotional Body

The emotional body is a very sensitive part of the Etheric anatomy. Its color is silver blue. It lies parallel with the physical body and should be the same size and shape. When raised, its position averages about ten to twelve inches above the physical body. Position may vary slightly. The body should be centered exactly with the physical body.

The emotional body displays several anomalies directly related to the emotional health of the client. Interestingly, in an emotionally sensitive person, or one who is not self-nurturing enough, or who is feeling isolated and alone, the emotional body will often swell up and become very soft. When the emotional body swells, the physical body may actually gain weight or look and feel puffy.

The emotional body may also become small and dense, with a sensation that it is too tight. This indicates that the client has a terrific amount of control issues or has instilled a lot of self-protection and there is practically no self-nurturing going on. This affectation may actually cause constipation and/or low physical and emotional energy levels. When the body is contracted, the internal energy becomes restricted and communications to, from, and throughout this body become restricted, as does the health of the emotional body and, in turn, the body of the physical.

This body may become blocked with dense areas of energy. These blockages can run the gamut in size or density. The dense areas are unacknowledged or unprocessed emotional experiences and feelings that have been hidden because they were too hard or the client did not have the skill to work through them. These blockages may cause physical symptoms, including acute or chronic pain, and can be found anywhere in this body. When they are found and released, the physical symptoms of pain or discomfort also disappear.

All of the Etheric bodies have external walls, a thin skin of energy that holds them together. Particularly, the walls of the emotional body can become damaged or torn for different reasons. When they do, the client may show symptoms in their 3–D experiences, such as malaise, lack of focus, fluctuating energy levels physically, and indecisiveness.

Affectations in the emotional body usually correlate with and validate what is found with the throat, solar plexus, and second chakra areas.

The Mental Body

The mental body is bright lemon yellow when it is healthy. It resides about ten to twelve inches above the emotional body. The mental body usually shows dysfunction when people are mentally stressed, have cyclic thinking that does not resolve, or have beliefs that are extremely strong and yet do not resonate as truth for the client.

Affectations in the mental body can profoundly affect the physical body. One of the first kinds of affectations we might find with the mental body is that it will become very inflamed, surrounded by red energy. When this happens, the client may feel unsettled, their life may have a lot of chaos in it, and things may go wrong a lot for them.

When reason or answers cannot be found for situations in the client's life experience, the mental body, may begin to armor itself. Its outer skin may become extremely dense to the point that energy flow in that part of the body may come to a complete halt.

The mental body may also display blockages to different degrees of size, depth, density, and location. Blockages in this body may also be directly related to physical pain or chronic problems that could not be found with normal medical testing.

The Intuitive Body

The color is bright white with a violet-colored mantle over the shoulder, back, and chest. This body resides ten to twelve inches above the mental body. The intuitive body does not usually show any blockages or injuries. When it does, the practitioner can just about bet that wherever the blockage is found in the intuitive body correlates with chronic problems or pain in the physical body. Once cleared in the intuitive body, the problem in the physical goes away.

The most common anomalies found with the intuitive body are misalignments or angulation off center. The body will tilt to varying degrees on its center axis. It may also slide off center with the physical body in either direction.

When used regularly, the intuitive body, looks generally normal. If it isn't being used, it may become smaller and somewhat denser. If the client has begun using their intuitive gifts or their Seventh Sense to any large degree, this body may actually expand and begin to glow very brightly. If it does, care must be taken to achieve balance of this body because any aspect of the Etheric anatomy that becomes overcharged can be as dysfunctional as if it were too small or undercharged. The system must have equality and balance; otherwise, different problems may occur.

The Causal Bodies

The causal bodies are very special in their placement and their importance. There are two of them, and they are positioned on either side of the centerline, away from the stack of other Etheric bodies. They are almost like Etheric ballast, anchoring the balance between our human selves and our connection with the divine. Our causal bodies used to be a calico set of greens, teals, and browns, but with the recent energy shifts that are taking place on universal and inter-dimensional levels, these bodies have begun to glow in new color harmonics that range from bright light teal to sea green. They are also no longer in a set center alignment and may float parallel above the other bodies in different positions of alignment in order to maintain balance during energy shifts.

The causal bodies are a harmonic octave point in our overall connection with creation. They are our oldest example of manifested being. Their position is dimensionally at the outer realm of formed mass and matter. Our causal bodies are our most ancient selves and representative of our very beginning as traveling souls from one lifetime to another.

The causal bodies are positioned left and right of center, representing our female and male aspects, respectively. When our causal bodies are out of alignment with each other or with our other Etheric bodies, we may struggle with our male or female aspects. For example, a woman may become angry or aggressive, or a man may struggle with ego issues or a sense of powerlessness. Symptoms can run the gamut, but it is on this level that changes can be made to restore inner balance for the client.

The causal bodies are almost never blocked, and again, if they are, the problem is longstanding, spanning many lifetimes, and most likely chronic. If a blockage or injury is found at this level, there is a good chance that the problem has been remembered within the overall energy field and has been suffered for multiple lifetimes.

One common kind of injury to these bodies that doesn't apply to the above is that the outer edges of these two bodies may become frayed or rough, feeling like they have minor tears. These bodies have been with us through every lifetime our souls have traveled and, so, may have become worn and torn from use. The outer edges of these bodies can be easily smoothed and repaired. When wear and tear exhibits on this level, it does not usually cause physical symptoms or even third-dimensional affectedness unless the injuries are severe.

The causal bodies may also reveal that a client has gifts that they are or are not using. These usually show up symbolically as something the bodies are wearing or carrying. We may not always be able to interpret what they mean, but we really don't have to. I usually tell a client that she has great gifts waiting to be discovered, but even if I receive an interpretation of what those gifts are, I don't give that information because discovering it is part of the client's journey.

The Body of the Soul

The body of the soul is bright white, almost transparent, and nearly always perfect in presentation. It is rarely damaged or blocked in any way. If it is, the injury is generally karmic or so severe in its physical representation that the issue is likely terminal or extremely debilitating. The body of the soul is about eighteen to twenty-four inches above where the causal bodies reside.

Generally, when working at this level, it is the energy field around the soul body that requires our attention, not the body proper. This field may become littered with old energies or blockages that represent karmic issues at play. If the blockage has no vitality and does not feel heavy or vital or even dense, the energy of this blockage is an old karmic instance that is long past and no longer applicable. It can be cleared from the field with no problem.

If the blockage has much substance or weight and feels very vital or emits a force of energy, it is a current karmic situation that is playing out in the client's life. These should not be cleared because they are part of the client's journey.

Sometimes this field becomes littered with little specks of what look like energetic dust. This is merely interference in the field that should be cleared. Once this is done, the soul has a clear view of its journey and can make excellent choices along the way.

The Physical Body

The physical body may show any types or kinds of affectations. It may have areas that are inflamed, dull, blocked, irritated, and dense. You name it; it might be found in the body physical. Amazingly, the physical body tells us a vast story about our client. Where we find anomalies has everything to do with the client's current and past life experience as well as his perceptions and views of it and his unresolved issues. Here are some of the most often found areas of information:

- **Soft spots just below the collarbone and on the chest, centered between the shoulder and breastbone**—These represent close relationships, usually of a romantic nature. The left is usually representative of a female person; the right, male. On occasion a very strong female may show up on the male side or a very effeminate male person may show up on the female side, but generally the sides represent the actual sex of the romantic partner.

- **Large groups of nerves pass through this area that can be causal to issues in the face, neck, shoulder, and arm**—These areas can be repaired energetically to alleviate pain that is being experienced. They may also lead to issues in other parts of the body. Clearing here will allow energies to flow more fully so that corrections happen elsewhere in the body as a result of the fuller energy flow. There may also be no physical pain in reference to unresolved relationship issues; instead, the pain or issues may be emotional in nature.

- **The solar plexus area**—Holds grief and unexpressed anger.

- **Bottom of the ribs**—Usually represents past or present difficulties with a sibling or child, a close relative, or even, in some cases, a friend. Left is female; right is male.

- **Left lower abdomen**—Represents unexpressed or unresolved mother issues.

- **Right lower abdomen**—Represents unexpressed or unresolved father issues.

- **Hips**—Flexibility about adjusting to experiences in the past.

- **Knees**—Sometimes past lives will be revealed at this point. Also about flexibility in general.

- **Feet and ankles**—Injuries and pain in these areas represent resistance to forward movement into a new situation.

- **Toes**—Worrying about details that are generally unimportant.

- **Hands**—Left represents receiving. If someone has not learned to receive easily in their life, there will likely be clogged points of energy on the hands and wrists. The right side represents giving. Someone who is either afraid to give of themselves or gives too much will likely have clogged energy points in the hand or wrist.

- **Fingers**—Can represent emotional issues, particularly about current circumstances in which a specific issue has arisen that may be causing worry or concern. The middle fingers may also indicate sexual anger or frustration.

- **Feet**—Can represent ignorance that led to a current situation.

The Body Tells a Story

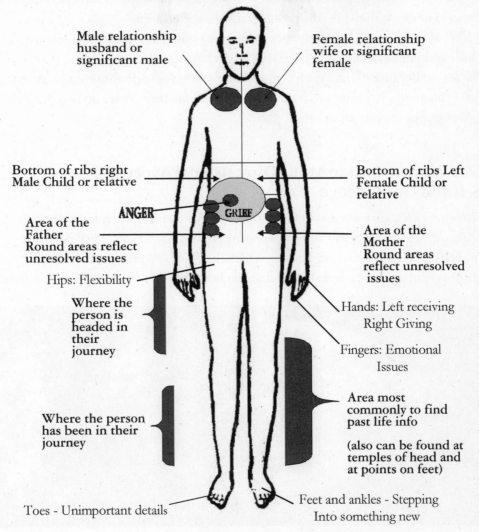

Male relationship husband or significant male

Female relationship wife or significant female

Bottom of ribs right Male Child or relative

Bottom of ribs Left Female Child or relative

ANGER

GRIEF

Area of the Father Round areas reflect unresolved issues

Area of the Mother Round areas reflect unresolved issues

Hips: Flexibility

Where the person is headed in their journey

Hands: Left receiving Right Giving

Fingers: Emotional Issues

Where the person has been in their journey

Area most commonly to find past life info

(also can be found at temples of head and at points on feet)

Toes - Unimportant details

Feet and ankles - Stepping Into something new

The organs and systems within the body physical each have their own unique harmonic makeup and can often be attuned to normal functioning. The overall body also has a unique harmonic make-up that becomes attuned in conjunction with the Etheric bodies. Specific work can be done with the physical body, but caution must be taken not to focus on the specific area so much as to find the actual cause. Sometimes the problem is being caused elsewhere, and repairing the area of cause alleviates the problem in its affected area.

What we must always remember is that the body is a cohesive and intricately choreographed system of energies that have come together to form the reality of the client. Because of that, each client's body will reveal different things. There is no set norm when it comes to multi-dimensional healing. Never do two people's systems appear exactly the same.

Our Connections to Multi-Dimensional Aspects of Self and Our Lineage

There are two large vortexes of energy that are extremely important in Etheric healing. They are a Yin and Yang, of opposite polarities, and connected deep into the body directly into the pranic tube, which then feeds the information into the chakras system where it is distributed throughout the body via the meridian system.

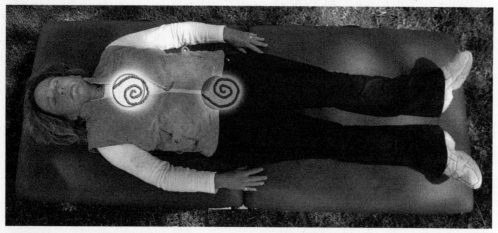

Two major vortexes are very important to us. The Yin, or high heart vortex, flows clockwise and is our connection with all of our other-dimensional aspects. Tracking the segments of this vortex can tell us where our aspects have fragmented out of alignment or have moved out of harmonic alignment. Usually those that have moved away from the straight alignment are relative to certain ages in our current life. The lower one, the Yang, which is between the solar plexus and the second chakra, flows counter-clockwise and brings us information from our entire lineage. Tracking the segments of this one can tell us where in our generational history dysfunction may have begun.

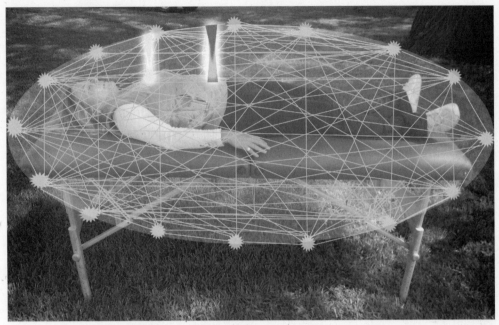

The two vortexes that feed us information about our other-dimensional aspects and
our lineage connect to the outer wall of our external field.

The Upper Vortex (Yin)—Our Other-Dimensional Aspects

In what we call the high heart area of the chest, a little bit above the physical
heart at the center of the chest and just a hair left of the center of the breast bone,
there is a vortex of immense strength that flows in a clockwise fashion from outer
dimensions into our bodies.

This vortex is light golden yellow in color and represents all of our multi-
dimensional aspects. Remember that we talked earlier about how we have aspects
of ourselves in all levels of reality, how those aspects can become fragmented
or out of alignment, and as a result, life can become difficult? It is by using this
vortex that we can track and realign those aspects. Our otherworldly aspects also
represent past, present, and future and may often represent particular ages when
we experienced trauma during our lives.

The vortex is positioned with its wide part down and its apex, or point, up. In
the same way that dimensions become lighter and lighter the farther out they

go, the vortex does too. The vortex comprises many little segments all strung together. Each segment is about an inch long. The segments organize widely at first, beginning at the bottom of the vortex and then become shorter, tighter, and closer together as the spiral of segments becomes smaller and smaller the farther out it goes. The closer to the bottom of the vortex a segment is, the more recent the time and age. For example, if we find a segment just an inch or so up the vortex, we can deduce by that positioning that the represented age is approximately fifteen years in the past. A segment another inch or so up the vortex likely represents another ten or fifteen years in the past and so on. Usually, in an adult we only need to assess about four to six inches of the vortex wall because beyond that we get out of the current lifetime. Most of the misalignments we find are caused during current life events and traumas. Sometimes an aspect moves out of alignment because it somehow represents an age, a set of traits, or an experience that the client doesn't accept about themselves.

For instance, when I first discovered this wonderful way of tracking time and age, I knew that I had something missing in my own alignment that I just couldn't seem to locate. There was a part of me that felt like an angry adolescent. Certain events or situations would trigger a very negative feeling in me that I didn't like at all. I went looking for that part, and when I finally found it, it was an aspect of me when I was sixteen years old, a very difficult and painful time in my life. I realized that every part of me had rejected myself in that time because I felt betrayed by those who supposedly loved me, and I did not feel as if I belonged anywhere. That feeling of aloneness and rejection was very painful. I felt damaged, imperfect, and rebellious, even angry. I really had to work at accepting that time in my life as part of my overall self and healthfulness, but when I finally did, my entire outlook and behavior in response to certain situations changed dramatically.

In order to track the multi-dimensional aspects of a client, we can simply take our hand and scan the segments one at a time around the vortex spiral. If a segment feels damaged, it likely represents a certain age or time when there was trauma in the client's life. Many of these traumas are found in childhood or at adolescent ages. Finding a damaged aspect, the healer can stop and experience the energy of that segment and may actually be able to intuit the age that the trauma occurred and even the kind of event.

A segment that is torn or feels detached represents an aspect that is partially or completely out of alignment. A detached or severely damaged segment also tells us that the event that caused the damage was likely a serious trauma to the client.

When an aspect of us is out of alignment, we no longer have a multi-dimensional connection with our other aspects beyond that point. In a way, a piece is missing from our lines of communication. Our perceptions and abilities to draw on our experiences actually become limited.

By repairing the damaged, torn, or separated segments along this vortex, we are, in essence, attuning all of a client's multi-dimensional aspects, past, present, and future. They become a finely tuned instrument that is at once cohesive and clearly communicating amongst all aspects. Achieving these repairs creates a great sense of inner balance in the client and also allows for easier access to both logical and intuitive clarity.

The Lower Vortex (Yang)—Our Lineage

Placed at the exact center of our abdomen between the solar plexus and the second chakra is another extremely powerful and important vortex. It is red in color and represents our lineage all through time. It rotates in a counter-clockwise manner, driving information about our entire lineage into our bodies.

Some Asian cultures, in particular martial arts, call this spot on our body the Dan Jun. In martial arts, the practitioner is taught to close off this vital area of energy too so that energy builds up in the body and then can be transferred by various movements in the martial arts cadences.

This vortex is segmented similarly to the upper vortex and can be evaluated and time tracked the same way. Only in this instance, each segment represents a generation. Segments that are damaged in this vortex will feel dark and powerless, low in vitality, torn, or damaged. They don't usually disconnect as the aspects do in the upper vortex.

Often somewhere in our lineage, dysfunction began and then became hereditary either as a behavior, pattern, illness, or dysfunction. For instance, some forms of abuse such as sexual abuse, mental instability, addictions such as alcoholism, or other inherited behaviors may run in families and can be traced back to the first ancestor who had the problem. Once disconnected from the lineage, the current problem may be more easily overcome if not eradicated altogether.

Certain behavioral patterns and dysfunctional patterns that began in a previous generation are usually learned, inherited as cellular memories that we picked up in utero, or inherited genetically. Once we repair the corresponding segment on the vortex wall, we forever break that hereditary patterning. When we do, if there are generations between our current life and the one that is repaired, they may also experience improvement or sudden awareness regarding past issues. The repair becomes a chain reaction that corrects past, present, and future simultaneously.

The Meridian System

The meridian system is a network of invisible pathways throughout the body through which energy flows. It is fed energy by the chakra system and kept in place by the electromagnetic fields of the chakras. There are many different meridian lines, and each has a set of functions and purposes regarding our general health as well as specific problems.

Along these lines, spaced in varying intervals, are little power points. If we looked closely at the meridian system it would look like an organized web of connect the dots.

Each point along every meridian line has a specific meaning and function related to the overall healthfulness of the body. Sometimes these little points become clogged, blocking the energy flow along the rest of that meridian pathway. At other times, they can become inflamed, or overcharged, causing a sequence of issues in the body that often leads to physical symptoms.

The energy that flows through the meridian system is the basis for acupuncture and has been evaluated and studied for centuries. It is used in Chinese medicine and many other Eastern applications. Working with the meridian points is a fine art that can relieve pain, cure illnesses, and help to prevent them too.

As I grew more confident with my strange but effective abilities in healing, I found my hands and fingers being guided to touch specific areas of the body. If my hands didn't move of their own accord, I actually began to see (and still do) little lights on the body. A red light meant inflammation, a yellow one meant that I needed to do specific work on that point, or to touch it in conjunction with another point, and a dark spot meant that the energy at that point was blocked to at least some degree.

When I saw the dots, I instinctively touched them one after the other with just a fingertip or two as if my hands were doing an Etheric dance. People loved to watch because it was beautiful and fluid, a strangely choreographed art coming directly out of the ethers. When I connected the points, energy began to flow more freely, to release, or to become unclogged. When the energy in one place changed, I noticed that it also changed in other parts of the body. My clients felt energy pathways open up and begin to move fluidly in different areas of their bodies.

I honestly had no idea of the significance of what I was doing back then, but I kept doing it because my client's bodies and energy fields were responding. I found that I nearly always touched, not only one point on the body, but as I did so I was making connections between two or more areas nearly all of the time. Sometimes I touched two or three or four points simultaneously and at other times even more.

My hands seemed to have minds of their own. I never questioned where they touched or why, I just let my guidance free flow. I began to suspect that what I was doing had something with the meridian lines, but to this day I have never studied them. Even though the information is easily available, I have trusted my cosmic connections and stayed out of my brain, letting my consciousness stream freely. Doing so has been extremely effective over the years.

I never really needed to know what was happening or what the little points all over the bodies meant, but I was a little curious. I had made a practice of not mentally questioning this strange healing process. Many of my experiences were so out of the ordinary, and yet so effective, that I didn't want to pollute them with brain stuff. I felt that I might begin to influence my gifts subconsciously if I believed that the process should go one way or another.

I was confirmed in my belief that I never needed to explore or mentally understand the details of the meridian system when I was on a teaching tour in New Zealand years ago. A Chinese acupuncture doctor attended one of my workshops there. Being a bit new at teaching my healing process back then and, honestly, a bit overwhelmed at everyone's responses to my work, I was still surprised by the reactions and opinions that came from those who encountered this powerful process.

One day during our class break, the acupuncture doctor approached me and asked me to work on his wife. Assuming at the time that this man likely knew much more about energy work than I did, I politely asked him why he didn't work on her. He told me that she didn't like needles, so he thought maybe I could help her. There was only one condition: He got to come and observe. Being very used to having people watch me work, I agreed.

At the appointed day and time, the doc and his wife came to meet me. I worked within the wife's energy field diligently and methodically with my usual rhythm. Each time I found any area of significance I silently gestured to the doc. He and I exchanged no words at all while I worked. After the session was over, I looked up and saw him shaking his head with a kind of strange look on his face.

"What is it?" I asked. Still finding my confidence back then, I was a little unsure of his reaction to what I had just done and I was honestly concerned that he didn't believe a thing (remember, I was very new at taking this whole thing public back then).

He didn't answer me and just kept shaking his head. Again, I asked the same question. Finally, he spoke.

"Who taught you?"

I reminded him that he had already heard my story in the class the day before and that the story was still true and hadn't changed since class.

Again, shaking his head, he asked me, "Who taught you?"

"I told you. Why?" I answered curiously.

"It was amazing," he said. Every time you touched an organ, you also touched its corresponding power point on the body. You went through the entire system and didn't make one mistake. Your acuity of the meridian system is impressive. How could you possibly know this? It takes years of study to be this proficient! Who taught you?"

Honestly, all I could do was laugh. My answer to him was simply "Well, at least now I have an idea of what I am doing!" I was secretly awed to hear this amazing validation of what was happening so naturally. Having had no prior knowledge of these points, I had allowed my intuition and Seventh Sense to afford me a purely cosmic education that was right on accurate!

He shook his head some more. It really was hilarious then and still is now. I realized years later that an important part of what I was doing was very similar and in some cases identical to acupuncture, only in a purer form and without needles. I began to understand why some of the things that my hands did were very important to the overall healing of the body. I discovered that the places I checked for balance were intersections of multiple energy lines and that by completing a circuit between them with my hands and fingers, my energy field was naturally evaluating, reading, and correcting that of my clients.

I also began to realize that I was naturally closing smaller circuits, allowing the energy in a specific area of the meridian line to expand, reach a climax, then spontaneously balance back into a normal flow and rhythm. Connecting multiple points also formed specific energy nets that changed larger areas.

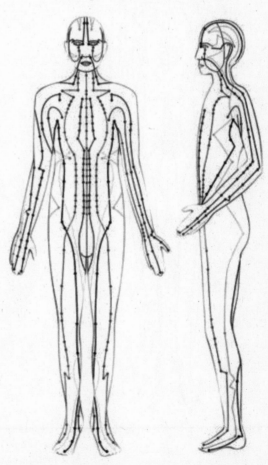

Since then I have had many acupuncturists in my classes who have switched to running energy the way I teach them and using fewer needles than they had previously. They find that the new way is, in some cases, even more powerful than using the needles and always at least as effective.

For me, learning all of those tiny points and their meanings by rote remains unimportant, at least for my purposes. I do, however, usually provide a set of charts in my class workbooks for curious students. I also have a great respect for the work of acupuncturists. It is a precise science and an effective method of healing as well as illness prevention.

The major meridian pathways in our bodies.

What I know without a shadow of a doubt is that the meridian system is a vital part of the overall energy system in conjunction with all the layers and levels of energy that compose us. Believe it or not, if allowed, the hands and fingers will go where the energy corrections are needed.

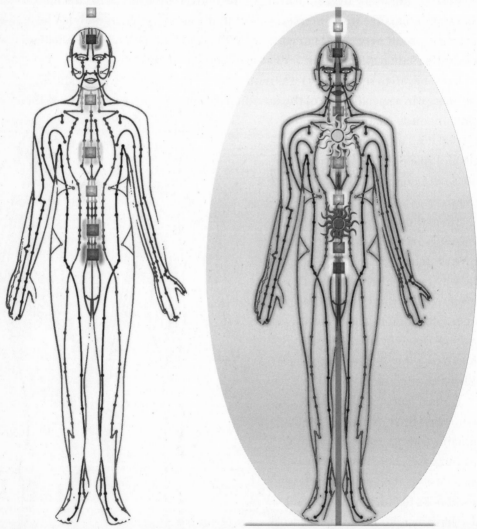

The Meridian System is fed by the chakras

The pranic tube feeds the chakras which then power the meridian system. The kundalini is a mixing system that maintains energy balance and flow. The larger vortexes at the high heart and mid abdomen connect us to our multi-dimensional aspects and our infinite lineage, respectively.

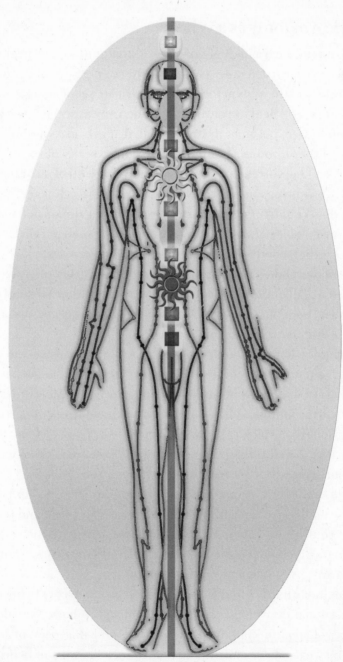

The energy system, with external field, meridian lines, chakras, and kundalini all together, gives us an idea of how all of these vital parts of our systems work together in a multi-layered process.

Our Etheric Anatomy as a Whole

Once we understand each aspect of our Etheric anatomy, we can begin to understand how each system, each layer, chakra, body, or energy pathway cooperates within the entirety of the system to create an intricate set of energies that nurture, feed, cleanse, and heal us continually. When any aspect or even a tiny area of our complete system becomes dysfunctional, it affects us as a whole.

Each of our Etheric bodies is connected through a series of vortexes that I described earlier. One vortex carries information about all of our Etheric aspects, while the other one brings us information about our entire lineage. These vortexes also serve to equalize energetic pressure from one dimension to the other, in the same way that black holes equalize pressure between parallel realities.

Each of our Etheric bodies are connected by these vortexes.

Every one of our bodies has a similar outer elliptical layer of protective energy and a grid system. All of these are connected into the greater fabric of creation. All of our bodies, both physical and Etheric, have other aspects. We are a system of being, not a singular reflection of creation.

Only our physical bodies have chakras because they are necessary to move the energy through our denser physical manifestations. All of our bodies have meridian systems that are similar in nature. We are amazing beings, able to draw from and contribute to the infinite. When we begin to assemble all of our parts, the total picture looks a lot like the picture below. To avoid visual chaos, I left out the meridian lines in the picture as well as the extreme higher and lower chakras, since we have not addressed them in regards to the basic healing format. You can still get a pretty good idea of just how complex we are and how far reaching our effect is within creation.

All of these bodies overlap within our soul groups and send and receive information to our soul families about how we can participate with each other to further the journeys of our souls. The kinds of challenges we desire, what we need, who we are in any given moment, the list goes on.

We are inevitably hard-wired within creation in a matrix of being that is more powerful and subtler that we ever could have realized. What we can do is unlimited. The forces of creation contain all possibilities and all aspects of anything and everything we need. Once we understand this, what we now believe to be miracles can become commonplace in our future.

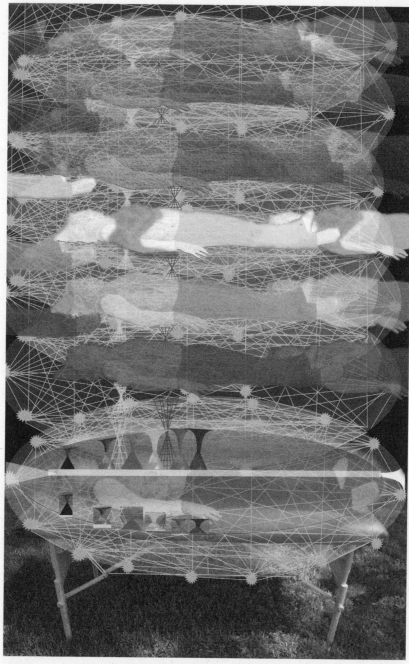

Our total Etheric anatomy as it is in Creation.

CHAPTER NINE

Things No One Wants to Talk About

The subjects in this chapter are compiled from some of my experiences. Everyone's Etheric anatomy is affected in different ways. Some of us may have similar harmonics or affectations that interfere with our systems, but no two are alike. There are times when we are more vulnerable than others. Emotional or physical trauma, being extremely overtired, drugs, alcohol, and even journeying out of body unprotected are just some of the ways that we may become open targets to taking on affectations in our energy fields.

Sometimes otherworldly influences can have a direct effect on our everyday lives. They come in all shapes and sizes and can create anything from subtle differences in our experiences to complete chaos. Even the very idea that some of these affectations might exist brings fear to many people. Hollywood has even made movies about some of them that are often exaggerated—but not always. This section addresses issues that do happen. The information here is more for awareness than anything else. A good practitioner of *Touching the Light* should have at least some knowledge of these subjects because encountering them cold with no prior knowledge of them can be mind-blowing to say the least! I don't expect anyone to run out and start finding these anomalies in everyone they meet. These are not found every day but can sometimes turn up when we least expect them.

It is important to remember that there is no reason to be afraid of any of them. Creation has infinite aspects of life that can influence us in our human form. Sometimes that life comes in forms that are so foreign or different from what we know that they are frightening, repulsive and even at times, downright terrifying. We are not the only living creatures and energy forms. Know that, in the same way that each of us is unique in all of creation, so are they. Each of them holds a vital part in the construct of creation just as we do. With this perception, we can approach a variety of strange and interesting subjects as observers rather than victims or participants.

I have chosen to break these anomalies into different categories and subcategories so that we can look at each in detail and, where appropriate, with greater explanations. When I hold seminars for learning my healing methods, I often add a bonus day for what I call "the weirdness."

On the morning of that day everyone tentatively comes into the room big-eyed, holding his or her breath, and wondering just what we will be talking about on that day. They want to know but are afraid to bring these creepy ideas into their realities. Before the day is over, though, everyone is having a great time and asking deep and well thought out questions.

What we must remember above all else is that when we work within the light and have instilled our protection in the manner we discussed earlier, none of these things can access our energy fields no matter what. As we explore this subject more fully, I will tell you a few stories. Some of them may sound as if they are out of a very good imagination or an intense sci-fi movie. I assure you that they are true, as are the details.

You can't catch anything by reading this chapter, honest. Nothing will jump off the pages and attack you or attach to your energy system. What you might catch is awareness about some very important issues that can and do affect some people. The main thing I want to stress in relation to this chapter is that dealing with these issues is not for an inexperienced practitioner, nor is it for anyone who has any fear whatsoever of the unusual or the unknown. Fear can get us into real trouble because some of these anomalies thrive on fear. This chapter is more of an FYI to the reader because most people won't talk about these subjects, and some who do propagate little information and a whole lot of fear.

Working inter-dimensionally can be full of surprises. We never know where a soul has been in its travels, how it may be affected or even who might have hitched a ride. Each and every person we work with has a different harmonic field and within that can be any combination of affectations. We don't need to get into drama and trauma or fear or any other big deal reaction to any of these things. What is important is to stay out of our heads, keep our cool, stay protected, and do whatever is necessary to assist the client.

I look at these subjects as anomalies in our systems, or beings that, for one reason or another, may be temporarily out of their own universal neighbor-hoods. We are a minuscule part of a greater creation, and within that creation are any number of kinds of beings and levels of consciousness. Some are harmonic with us and some aren't. Some of these anomalies are minor to moderate in how they can affect us, while others are the things nightmares are made of. Either way, only a very experienced, fearless, open-minded, and confident practitioner should ever do some of the things you are about to read about. So relax, keep breathing, and keep on reading.

Cords and Reasons for Them

What are cords and where do they come from? The cords that attach in the pelvic area or in the mid-back are usually instilled upon others by people who connect to them in unhealthy ways. Co-dependent, abusive, or controlling relationships very often create unhealthy cords between the participants. This is usually some-thing that neither the attacher nor the attachees, so to speak, are even aware of. Sometimes cords are inflicted intentionally too.

Etheric cords are unhealthy connections between two or more people. They can also be self-inflicted, connecting some of the Etheric bodies to the physi-cal world. Usually, cords attach in one of two places: either the pelvic area, or the center of the back. They can also be found connecting the physical, emotional, or mental bodies together in an inflexible attempt to control different aspects of these three bodies.

For example, someone who does not trust his emotions may have inadver-tently instilled cords between his emotional and mental bodies in an attempt to rationalize his feelings. Someone who completely overthinks everything may have created ties between the physical and emotional bodies in a self-defensive attempt to control them. Of course, the control is an illusion, but the self-defensive gesture is very real.

Cords can be gotten during sex, when deep connections are made between two people or one of the two who are involved latches onto the other person energetically.

When instilled intentionally, energetic cords are used to control people, to drain their energy to the benefit of the other. Strangers almost never attach cords to us. They are nearly always relative to someone we know or have known.

Cords attach with a root-like appendage that is a lot like a taproot. The root actually burrows down into the energy field of its victim and latches on deep in the field. In addition to the taproot, some cords have multiple roots that spread out into the energy field after the main root attaches.

Locating and reading cords is not hard to do. The more recent the cord, the more vital it is. A recent cord will look or feel like a live umbilical cord, vital with blood flow. Usually, recent or current cords look like inflamed tissue that ranges in color from pink to shades of purple, as if the tissue isn't getting enough oxygen. A recent cord is vitally alive and very warm as a rule.

Left of center in the low pelvic area represents the female. If a cord is found in this area, the person who has attached it is usually someone of female gender. When found to the right of center, cords have generally been instilled by a male person. Sometimes one or the other crosses the centerline. This might happen in the case of, for instance, a female with a lot of male tendencies, or a male who is very effeminate, but this is a good rule of thumb. So if we were to find a cord in the lower right pelvic area of a woman, chances are that it is relative to a male person with whom she has had some sort of relationship. The more vital the cord, the more recently it has become attached.

Someone who has some sort of an agenda regarding the victim usually instills cords that are found in the mid-back. When found in the mid-back, the cords are draining energy out of the system. This is a type of psychic attack. A psychic attack is when one person sends negative (usually) energy at another person on Etheric levels. Being hit by the energy of another, especially when their intentions are anything but good, can even be painful. When a cord attaches as a result of a major psychic attack, our 3-D world can become inflammatory and chaotic and nothing works the way we normally expect. We become moody, and our energy levels, both physical and emotional, are inconsistent. We may even become angry or depressed for no apparent reason.

A cord can remain attached even after the death of the one who inflicted it. They can also remain with our light bodies and carry through with an energy system from one lifetime to another, even into multiple incarnations. Cords that are older, from previous lifetimes, are shrunken, shriveled, and gray or brown. They have no vitality and look like small, withered, old branches that have rotted and decayed. These older cords are not harmful, but they can continue to contribute to minor to moderate energy loss in a person's system.

Removing Cords

Cords should never be left in place when they are found. They can be found by using the hand to scan the energy in the pelvic and mid-back areas. Cords feel like an interruption in the energy field. They may feel different than the rest of the field. They may feel more intense or like a blank spot or an area that is very cold. If the cord is recent and very active, it might feel like a hot or very warm area, as you might imagine inflammation would feel.

Symptoms of cording are easy to recognize. Here are the main ones:

- Fluctuations in physical, mental, and emotional energy for no apparent reason.

- Difficulty concentrating.

- Inability to make decisions.

- Mild to moderate depression (from draining resources).

- May even cause irrational thinking about a person long after the relationship has ended. Can't let go of them even when they are destructive.

The process of removing a cord can be described as psychic surgery. The area of the energy field where the cord is attached must be laid open to reveal the roots of the cord. Directing an intention to the client's energy field to open around the root of the cord can do this.

Remember, in those moments we are merged within the field, so all we need to do is command that field to open where we need it to, and it will. Next, grab hold of the cord and gently twist it back and forth much like you are pulling a carrot out of the ground. Never yank on it because if the roots are broken off in the field, the cord can actually grow back. When you have loosened the cord enough by twisting it back and forth and slightly pulling, it will pop right out.

Once the cord is dislodged, it is very important to transmute the roots into inert matter. This is just another term for cosmic dust. Once the roots are destroyed, the cord can never reattach. It is best to transmute the energy of the cords into source light. This can also be done by intention, and you will feel the cord dissolve.

Someone else's cord won't attach to you or anyone else. They are only intended or instilled in a specific energy field, so there is no reason to worry about them attaching to you.

Implants

Implants are very real. There is a huge amount of speculation as to their source, ranging from any number of conspiracy theories to alien abduction. Their purposes can be as a tracking device; a system monitor that collects data about body functioning, genetic information, and responsiveness; to adjust the energy field of the host; or to transmit and receive information to and from the host.

Implants are most commonly found in the soft tissue of the head and ears; nasal passages; inside the sinus cavities; in the arms, wrists, and hands; occasionally in the legs and ankles; and inside the torso. Locations can vary depending upon the purpose of the implant.

There are many different kinds of implants and many different reasons for them. They range from being made of pure energy to what we call *hard copies*, little tiny mechanisms that seem to be made of some sort of metal or other material.

Some implants are quite fascinating because, once placed in a body, they actually morph to match the tissue they are planted in. They will become not only adapted to surrounding tissue, but also so closely similar in nature that they become virtually undetectable by normal medical means.

Hard Copies

Hard copies, when implanted in soft tissue, such as the ears or back of the head, can be felt most of the time and may make their wearer itch like crazy in that specific spot. They may also put off heat intermittently. They may be in the form of tiny disks, miniature bullet shapes, elliptical, or irregular in shape.

Dr. Roger Leir is well known in UFO circles for having removed many of these kinds of implants. He has had some analyzed, and to put it mildly, they are created of materials not of our world.

I have seen videos Dr. Leir has taken of procedures during which the implants moved position to avoid being taken out. One of his stunning videos shows an implant moving away from the scalpel and crawling under the skin up the patient's arm, presumably to avoid removal.

Dr. Leir found that if an implant is removed and stored in alcohol, formaldehyde, or other preservative, it will more often than not wilt away and virtually disappear or at the very least shrink and lose shape. Dr. Leir further discovered that, when removed, these kinds of implants are best stored in a sample of the patient's blood serum. When stored in this fashion, the implants will remain in their normal state.

Speaking of adapting, hard copies will also very closely mimic cartilage particularly in the *pinea*, the larger, flat, outer parts of our ears. The implant burrows into the cartilage and becomes so similar in its adaptation that the only way to surely remove it is to remove a great deal of the cartilage too. Of course this greatly disfigures the ear.

Most of the implants that have been removed and later analyzed have proven to be made of materials that are not from Earth. They are of metals or alloys that are foreign to us.

Actual removal of hard copy implants is not our job as alternative. If the client desires this, due to the strange and unpredictable nature of these little critters, a qualified medical person should do the procedure. There are few physicians who will take this subject seriously though. We can, however, disengage the tiny electronics or circuitry in this kind of implant so that they no longer work. Doing so is simple: as once an implant is located, we can tune into its harmonics and then introduce frequencies though our hands that are disharmonic to the implant and completely fry their mechanisms. I have had excellent success with disengaging implants with this method.

Etheric Implants

Etheric implants are made of pure energy and are often found in the chest, midbody, or abdomen. I have also found these on the soles of people's feet. I actually thought that placing them there had been quite clever because it isn't a place we would usually look for implants.

At first when I discovered Etheric implants, I wondered if I was imagining them until one day, as I removed one, I watched in awe as another one materialized in exactly the same place I had just removed the first one. Etheric implants are most often combinations or variations of yellows and or light greens in color and are usually but not always disk-shaped. The size of the disk can vary from about one to four inches in diameter. They can also be shaped like flat disks or like cylinders.

Etheric implants seem to have multiple purposes and functions, depending upon their locations in the body. Often they are placed at specific angles of fifteen or thirty degrees. I have found a few that are implanted at forty-five-degree angles as well. Those placed in the chest or upper torso are usually the larger ones. They seem to monitor body functioning and also gather data of different kinds from the body as well as the experiences of the host.

How we remove an Etheric implant is similar to how we disengage the hard kind, but in this case, we use energy to disband the particles that the implant is made of. We create energy that is disharmonic to the implant. As the new energy flows into the implant, the particles that the implant are made of become non-cohesive and come apart, rendering the fragments useless. Disbanding the particles is like taking the implant apart at its most basic level. Once disbanded, the particles are no longer cohesive and spontaneously return to basic light energy. Any particles that remain with the body automatically transmute to match the body harmonics in a normal energetic state. The process is fascinating to watch and easy to accomplish.

Spirits

Spirits are souls who have left their earthly bodies but for some reason have not moved on in their natural transitional process. Usually, they stay in places that are familiar to them or that have meaning, such as their home or where they died. Some spirits can attach themselves or their energy to a live person. Sometimes they do this because they feel that person has something they need, or perhaps there is something with the live person that needs to be resolved.

Spirits remain for a number of reasons. Some don't realize that they have died. They are confused and don't know to cross over into the light. Others have an agenda about something that they feel they must accomplish before they can cross over into the light. Some spirits are stuck for one reason or another and don't know how to move on. Sometimes there is such a bond between the departed and someone on earth that the departed spirit won't cross over because they want to keep an eye on, or stay as near as possible to, their loved one. There are also spirits who are held back from crossing over by the sheer grief of those who are left behind. Intense and long lasting, or unprocessed, grief can pull at a spirit and keep it earthbound. Some spirits are angry and can wreak havoc, making noises, moving objects, even furniture, and affecting electronics too.

Most spirits are quite harmless. Some are actually helpful to the living. They may even act as protectors or as Etheric guides. These spirits have already crossed into the light but have remained close by Ethereally. Most often when spirits are nearby or enter a room, there is a cold feeling in the immediate area. Sometimes the temperature in the entire room drops more than a few degrees. Some spirits are accompanied by a familiar smell, such as their perfume or, if a man smoked, the smell of his pipe burning. The accompanying smells will always be something that pertains personally and specifically to the spirit when it was alive.

When some spirits are near us, they actually feel so familiar that we can recognize who they are. We may also feel their emotions. Some can feel very intense, anxious, or chaotic. Some feel like pure love while others feel very sad. The emotions of spirits can truly run the gamut. Those who are sensitive to the presence of spirits often feel what the spirits feel, their emotions, their fears, and even at times their confusion.

Spirits may appear visually or energetically as nebulous forms of energy. They can often be seen with the naked eye. They may show up in photographs as wisps of smoky-looking photo anomalies or as orbs.

When we can see them, if their death was natural and uneventful, spirits will usually appear as they normally did or sometimes as what they believed to be their most perfect selves, younger or healthier. If the death was traumatic or sudden, and the spirit has not yet crossed into the light, the spirit may appear, injuries and all, until they come to grips with their new circumstances. Once they do, they begin to look more and more normal. I have seen spirits in many different ways, such as spectral forms, maybe missing part of their body, or so transparent they are barely visible, and I have seen them appear so strongly that they startled me because they look uncannily normal and solid in their appearances as if they were still alive.

In an effort to pursue unfinished business, spirits can attach to people or objects such as personal items or even a piece of furniture, haunting them until their tasks are achieved.

Sometimes in an effort to make contact, a spirit will touch a living person. This touch can be so real it is startling! I have felt this touch many times in countless places, particularly those of a historic nature, but it can happen anywhere. I have felt the spirits of little children tugging on my clothes to get my attention. Adult spirits often touch us in more meaningful ways.

My friend Van passed away several years ago. We had been best friends for nearly thirty years. She became acutely and seriously ill, and at the time, I was living across the country from her. I was frantically trying to make flight reservations to go and be with her at the hospital when I felt her leaving. Death was calling my friend, and I knew that she was resisting her transition, waiting for me to arrive. She knew that I would be able to take care of everything and assist her children with their loss.

I immediately picked up the phone and called the hospital. After a brief run around, I commanded that the phone be brought to my dearest friend. She was in a coma by then, but I knew without a doubt that she would hear me. The phone was put to her ear and I told her that I was on the way, I would be there soon and that I would take care of everything and everyone. I passionately told her that she was doing a terrific job, to just let go and go on. When I told her this, she tried to communicate with me on the phone but couldn't make the words happen. She was too weak, but without a doubt I know she not only heard me but also understood me. Shortly after we hung up she died. As she began her otherworldly journey, she traveled the miles between us in the blink of an eye. As I looked up from my laptop, she stood in front of me with a huge smile on her face and then, slowly, her smile never wavering, she vanished.

I flew all night and the next morning arrived at my friend's home. Her family was devastated at this unexpected event, as was I. There had been no warning at all. We were all very close, having shared many, many life events over the years. Together we planned her service. As a licensed minister, I was tapped to preside over the ceremonies. I wanted her memorial service to be the best and fullest expression of the way she lived her life as possible. Her kids wanted to make a power point presentation of her life to be on display at the service. They were having problems finding enough photos and I knew that Van had lots of great ones on her computer. I went to her home alone that evening both to get a little space to experience some of my emotions privately and to search her computer for the best images of Van.

Her computer was a dinosaur and everything I did took an excruciating amount of time as the pages loaded. I sat there waiting for a CD to burn and suddenly the air around me changed. Coming from behind me, I felt an unmistakable hand lay on each of my shoulders, warm and sure in their touch. I felt the fingers curl around the fronts of my shoulders, firming the grip, and I felt energy begin to come from the hands.

I immediately recognized Van's touch because for years, she had worked on my neck and shoulders to help me with a chronic neck issue. She always began by slowly and deliberately putting her hands on my shoulders. She would connect and then let this amazing energy flow from her hands into my sore muscles. It was this sweet touch that I felt. It was so sure, so real, there was no mistaking what was happening. What transpired next was even more amazing.

Her hands slid off my shoulders and her arms wrapped around me in the most loving hug I have ever felt in my life. My dear, dear friend was telling me she was okay and that she loved me. And then she was gone. Later I found out that her daughter had had a similar experience. Over the next few days there were little signs that Van was still there. I was cleaning out her bookshelves when suddenly an engraved rock that I had given her flew out of nowhere. It had been part of a set I had and she loved it so I gave it to her. A small insignificant thing but she wanted to return it. It flew straight out from a different shelf than the one I was working on, hit me (not too hard), and fell to the ground. I just laughed and said thanks.

After a few other touching moments, Van moved on in her journey not long after that, and I was happy that she did.

Often spirits will attend their funerals or memorial services before they move on. They even talk and attempt to interact with the guests and family members. My dad's funeral was no different. He passed away three days after the attack on the World Trade Center. He was in a different state from where I lived, so getting there in all the confusion and chaos was a challenge. There had been talk of martial law and curfews, and I was worried that I might not be able to get back home. I went anyway, of course.

As the funeral home filled, there were a huge number of attendees. Dad had been pretty prominent in his community for many years. There were a lot of people in attendance who I was surprised to see. Some were competitors and others that dad had fallen out with over the years. There was some real honoring of dad, and at the same time, a lot of empty words were spoken. Someone had cornered me and was going on about my loss (how could they have possibly known how I felt in that moment?), and all of a sudden, I felt someone tug my arm very hard in the direction of the exit door. I turned, startled, and no one seemed to be there. Then it happened again only harder, and I got it.

"Dad, this will be over soon," I promised, "then we can all leave." He tugged again but not quite as intensely.

"Really, Dad, I can't leave yet. These people are here for you, and as your eldest child, I need to be here." I felt him move back some, still present, watching impatiently. Patience never was one of dad's greatest virtues!

Some spirits remain because they are angry or intensely sad. These emotions can be extremely intense and are either about the circumstances of their deaths or specific situations or people who were in their lives on earth.

When a spirit attaches to a living person, they feed off of her energy, gaining strength and becoming more powerful. A person who has a ghost attached to her will often feel extraordinarily drained or exhausted. She might feel the emotions of the spirit, which can at times be overwhelming. She may also experience missing or moved items. An attached spirit can wreak havoc on a person's life, causing chaos and problems that can run the gamut. Having a ghost attached is not a good thing at all.

Sometimes a haunted place is nothing more than a curiosity or a nuisance, as footsteps or noises can be heard, or things may go missing or be misplaced. Some ghosts love to play games by stealing items and then later placing them somewhere they don't belong. We don't always know that spirits are present. Sometimes live human beings cohabitate with spirits and never even know.

A ghost can be detached from a living person in several ways depending upon the situation. Sometimes there isn't a relationship between the ghost and the living person at all, and the attachment is a matter of convenience for the ghost to draw energy. Spirits need to be guided to the light. Sometimes they just don't realize where to go.

At other times, they will not go into the light because they have an agenda. Of course, we don't want them attached to us day and night, disturbing our lives. Sometimes we can help them leave by helping them solve their dilemmas. Other times, they are determined not to leave until some problem is solved or an event takes place. Sometimes they don't want someone in their home or other particular place that was important to them.

When they are very determined, spirits may attach to our energy fields, draining us and causing problems in our everyday lives. A spirit can be detached from an energy field. Doing so requires re-harmonization of the living person's energy field so that the spirit is no longer able to harmonize with it and, therefore, can't remain attached.

Spirits can hear us and can be communicated with. Most of them simply need to cross over into the light. If there is resistance, we can assist them by communicating with them honestly and without fear. In cases when they don't know they have died, sometimes just giving them a little bit of education will be all they need. Others that are more resistant may need more than just information in order to depart. Sometimes they just need to say goodbye. Others have something important to convey or do. Each circumstance is individual in its needs and situation, so simple common sense is the best approach.

The important thing to remember is that ghosts are nothing to fear. They are just misplaced, disembodied people who sometimes need a little assistance to move along in their journeys.

Poltergeists

An unusual phenomenon that occurs and is linked to the spirit category is poltergeist activity. There are conflicting opinions about what causes this intense and often frightening phenomenon. When poltergeists are active, their actions can vary in type and intensity. Objects will fly across the room only to be broken or shattered. Furniture may be moved. Electrical appliances may seem to run of their own accord, and electronic devices such as TVs and stereos may turn off and on or play otherworldly messages.

Poltergeist activity most often is targeted at one person in the household, usually an adolescent girl, but it can affect everyone who lives there. I have also seen small children affected by a poltergeist.

Poltergeists have been known to inflict bodily harm in the form of scratches and bruises and causing falls or other "accidents" that lead to injury. Often with this kind of activity there are unexplained noises, voices, and messages that appear to be threatening.

I have noticed poltergeist activity is usually accompanied by an open portal to other dimensions somewhere in or about the location. Portals are inter-dimensional doorways that open and close depending upon universal positioning and influences like energy harmonics and polarities. Because of the nature of movement of creation (it actually pulses and moves slowly, changing position constantly) portals don't always access the same levels of reality.

There are times when portals become stuck in an open position for some reason or another. When that happens, entities and beings in other realities can find this open door into our reality. Sometimes this isn't a good thing or even a pleasant one. To me, poltergeist activity is most closely described as an inter-dimensional affectation. For some reason when the inter-dimensional portal is left open and beings enter into our world unseen but still affecting us, they have been attracted by the energy harmonics or a set of circumstances of a person or group of people.

Getting rid of poltergeists can be tricky because they don't necessarily want to go. In order to stop their influence, we must get them to go back into the portal and then close the aperture behind them. Working against poltergeists is not for the faint of heart nor the fearful. They can be dangerous, and they gain strength from emotions like fear. They feed on fear.

Imprints

Another form of spirit is not actually a presence. It is one whose energy has imprinted in the electromagnetic field at the moment of a severe trauma or a highly emotional or intense circumstance. Imprints are virtually ethereal recordings of the energy of specific situations and are harmless. An imprint of an emotionally intense moment can be indelibly left in the ethers for all eternity. As happens when we record onto a cassette tape, the moment of intensity is captured in the light of the fabric of creation as a record of that event.

Imprinted ghosts or spirits will repeat the same actions over and over again as if the moment had been caught in an endless loop. A great example of this is when we experience groups of Civil War soldiers who can be seen marching at certain times on certain days, appearing seemingly out of nowhere and then disappearing in the same way. They can be seen marching along, coming out of nowhere, then vanishing after a short time.

There are also ghost trains reported that come steaming out of the ethers, moving a short distance, then vanishing. Other events may be imprinted as well, such as a woman looking hopefully out of an upstairs window. The emotion of her longing for her long lost love was so intense that it was recorded in the electromagnetic field for eternity. Another example is the spectral form of a woman who appears on a stairway over and over again. She is seen in a flash from the waist up and then, as if she has suddenly had an idea or heard someone call her, she turns and vanishes. At another historic place we may hear footsteps at exactly the same time every day and see no one. We may see or hear a group of men discussing strategy plans from the time of the Civil War.

Imprints are fascinating and not at all dangerous. Their appearance can be intense for someone who has never experienced them before. Sometimes the imprints are in the form of voices, parts of a conversation, or the sound of footsteps that wander a certain area of the house night after night, beginning at exactly the same time each night.

Walk-ins, Assimilations, Star Walkers, and Reptilians

This category of weirdness contains several different life forms. These affectations are more rare than all the others we will be discussing, but they do exist. It is important that the reader not go away from this book believing that the following circumstances affect the general population. These instances occur in maybe one percent of the total population, but when they do, they are huge in effect and are very powerful in different ways.

Walk-ins

A walk-in happens when one disembodied soul takes over the living body of another. This might occur when the consciousness of a person has become so open and unprotected that it becomes available to almost any kind of being who decides to jump in. More often than not though, a walk-in occurs when someone is in the process of dying or is mortally injured. At the time of the dying or injury, a new soul takes over the body. Sometimes the walk-in actually pushes the too open or weakened consciousness out of a body and takes it over completely. In every case, a walk-in generally is not borrowing the body; it is literally stealing the body of another soul.

After a walk-in takes over, the body still looks like the person who used to occupy it, but often the new soul makes drastic changes to hairstyle, wardrobe, likes and dislikes, preferences, and pretty much everything about life in general. Demeanor usually changes and facial expression is often quite different. The body may gain or lose a large amount of weight.

A walk-in may or may not remember anything about the previous soul's life, including family members, spouse, and children. Sometimes there is residual memory so the adapting is a bit easier.

It is not unusual for a walk-in to be extremely angry, argumentative, or quite different from the person who used to inhabit the body. Generally, the original soul is no longer present. Usually a walk-in is human in nature, but I did meet one who was definitely not from around here!

I was having my usual Wednesday night meeting at my home, and a regular attendee brought a guest who was staying at her place. When they walked in, I immediately knew something was wrong. The woman started toning loudly and throwing energy at other people in the room. Her energy field was chaotic, and her facial expressions were not typical of a well-balanced human being. She was trying to "heal" everyone and not with their permission. This wasn't just someone with good intentions; this was way over the top!

A few questions from me to my friend brought the realization that the woman she had brought had recently been a prominent psychologist in her area. She was well known and had worked with many celebrities. Apparently, the woman had been working to open her consciousness more fully, and during one of these sessions with herself she began to vibrate severely. This kind of intense vibration can occur when another soul or consciousness enters a body. The woman had shaken so hard that she ended up on the floor. During this experience, the new soul, or being, entered her body.

Suddenly this prominent psychologist was no longer herself. The new being walked away from her lifelong practice and gave away all of the woman's belongings. From there, it took her out on foot away from her previous life and in search of who knows what. Remarkably, she landed a state away at my house.

The woman walked over and got right in my face, challenging every statement I made, telling me that my perceptions were all wrong and that she and only she was right. She was unwavering. It was creepy how close she got into my space, and her energy field was bizarre. We were practically nose to nose. I asked her not to direct energy at me or anyone who hadn't asked for it. She didn't appreciate my request at all. It was like she was on a mission. This walk-in was not one you would want as a friend. She was so intense it was uncomfortable. I couldn't imagine what the body was going through.

Her energy felt as if it was maybe inter-galactic or other-planetary, not like a normal human energy field. She was extremely disruptive and getting worse by the minute.

Often spirits and other worldly beings are attracted to light workers like moths to a flame because they recognize the source energy we work with. They also sometimes think we can help, but this one didn't want our help at all.

I have to be honest and say that at first I didn't have a clue what was going on with her, but then it hit me. She was a very "fresh" walk-in and hadn't adjusted at all to her new body and surroundings. Not, I might add, that she wanted to. She was on a mission but wasn't coherent enough to communicate it. Sometimes it takes a while for a walk-in to adapt, especially when it is a total takeover.

I have actually known several walk-ins through the years, and most of them adapt pretty well, but sometimes they get fixated on a person, place, or activity.

One walk-in that I knew had been a pretty well-rounded person with a consistent job and a fairly normal life. She was another one who allowed her consciousness to get too open with no protection or discernment as to the kinds of energies she was attracting and allowing into her body. One day someone took her over, and the change in her was night and day incredible. She began dressing only in black, lost an immense amount of weight, and became very needful and at the same time extremely assertive. She fixated on one particular person and wouldn't let up.

Treating her like her old self was completely ineffectual. She did not seem to have the synapses to follow general logic and boundaries. Finally, one day I had a talk with her regarding the changes I noted. I talked to her about walk-ins, and she immediately realized that was her circumstance. She finally balanced out over the years but never in any way close to who she had been originally.

A walk-in situation cannot be undone or "cured" if the new soul has taken over completely. Sometimes the original soul remains "in there" somewhere but is dominated by the new entry. In those cases, what can be done is to assimilate the two together harmonically so that they function as one and are more able to adapt.

Because of the hold the newer soul has on the body, it cannot be removed without doing grave damage to the body. The new soul has entered the body and filled it with its consciousness, so removing it would actually kill the body. If life force is taken from any of us, we will die. The same goes for walk-ins.

Interestingly, when we look ethereally at a body that has more than one soul, we may see one or the other in spirit form riding the body in tandem with the original soul.

Star Walkers

Another kind of walk is a lot different than what I have just described. I call this *assimilation*. There are what I call Travelers who can deconstruct their form and travel within the construct of creation or through wormholes to other realities and locations. When they come to Earth, often they will jump into a body, riding in simultaneously with the original consciousness much like a hitchhiker but always with a purpose. Usually, they will choose someone with a very open consciousness who is also a very strong person. At the time of entry, the body vibrates intensely to the point that it feels as if it may come apart. Then the star walker enters and joins with the original soul.

The feeling at first is like being tiny in relation to the new life force that has entered. It is as if the star walker is hovering above the original soul and often seems massive in size. A person who has had a star walker enter suddenly finds new gifts or knowledge or both.

For instance, someone may all of a sudden have knowledge of sciences they never knew about. They may instantly understand and be able to apply harmonics that are complex and rarely accessed let alone understood. Comprehension of energy comes as an added bonus with the addition of a star walker, and almost always these beings come into our world with a positive purpose to assist us with something, or to contribute technologies or information that can change how we do things.

The star walkers are peaceful beings and mean no harm. Sometimes they join a body just for a temporary time; at other times, they assimilate with the original soul into one consciousness that maintains the memories of the original soul along with the new information that the star walker has brought. Assimilation is usually done with the permission of the host person. This isn't necessarily a bad thing as nearly all-star walkers are peaceful beings with a positive purpose, and the information they carry becomes part of the consciousness of the host. Once assimilated, there is no way to tell one from the other as their energies are so well harmonized that no individuality remains.

Interestingly, a star walker can be brought forward and talked to or will channel through the host person. When they do this, the state of reality of the host person can become very fragile or completely overridden for that time.

One such being that I talked with communicated mostly in galactic symbols, but managed to give this fragmented explanation of his purpose. Here are his exact words:

> Not incarnated.
> Just to be.
> Structure in form.
> Listening.
> Answers come.
> Waiting, waiting.
> Here now, here now.
> Blended, we are.
> 2 total 1.
> Crystallized, emphasized.
> Time now, timeless.
> Feel, not words.
> My strength, your heart.
> Round, surround.
> Shifting time.
> Jonas, I am.
> None saved.
> My turn.
> Walk now.
> Flight.
> Freedom coming.

Must help.

2 dozen.

2 told.

To be just to be.

No fear divided.

Calm.

2 tone.

Arcturas.

Want answers, we have.

Numbers by 3s.

Win.

Charged, banded.

Positive charges.

Mysteries we share.

We share.

We share.

Jonas.

We are Jonas.

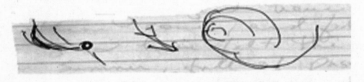

Drawing by Jonas explaining how he changed form to pure energy and entered our solar system. On the left we see him flying through the ethers. The middle is his form changing just before he enters our solar system. The right is our solar system.

Basically, he was telling me that he had waited a long time to come and that his purpose was entirely peaceful. He had come by way of Arcturus, where there is an intergalactic junction in the wormhole system. He spoke of his energies and form and how they had come together with his host. He didn't want anyone to be afraid. He was desperate to help some others of his group. Jonas had an amazing command of subtle energies and was very helpful to his host in teaching the host how to run energy through the body and change frequencies of that energy for purposes, such as healing or balancing an environment.

I later looked up the meaning of his name (pronounced John' us with a short o) and it means "the dove."

When a non-assimilated star walker and its host are on the healing table, it is possible to access each of them individually to converse. Once the star walker has been present in the body with the host for a while, it becomes more and more assimilated and harmonic with the host's energy field, and therefore, it becomes more difficult to see or access them separately. It may be necessary to assist with an assimilation to help the host being with functionality. To do this is to carefully and gently harmonize their fields of energy together, thus alleviating the duality and creating a singular consciousness and energy field.

Are There Really Reptilians?

Oh, yes, there are! I have seen three different types of reptilians, and none of them are desirable. When a reptilian enters into a host body, it assimilates just enough not to be obviously noticed, but there are telltale signs.

Someone who has a reptilian onboard has a certain something in their eyes that is at once captivating and repulsive. The eyes narrow and their gaze is usually quite direct. If one is sighted at all, a reptilian may momentarily reveal itself by turning its eyes completely red. To see this can be extremely unnerving.

Reptilians are nasty creatures of varying degrees of negativity. One type isn't quite as destructive but can cause all manner of problems in a person's life. They will run off everyone who is close to the host and attract people with less than good intentions. Relationships in general are nearly impossible for any long term because the energy of the reptilian invader is hard to be around for very long. They are deceitful, uncompassionate, and often abusive or mean spirited. They are also extremely manipulative and can make a human being do their bidding at will. Nothing a reptilian wants a person to do is ever likely to be a good thing.

Reptilians will enter a body without permission during times of open consciousness or inebriation from alcohol or drugs. They love people who are weak in conviction and personality, and they feed off of negative emotions.

The least nasty of these creatures is actually kind of beautiful in appearance. At least its scaly skin is. Its entire body is covered in scales that are opalescent, reflecting the light to change colors in ranges of light greens, silvers, blues, and teals. They are built very stocky with massive thighs and chest as well as upper arms. Their faces are kind of flattened with a low wide nose and their eyes are beady and kind of golden-colored with flecks of orange. The best way I can describe how one of these guys works is to tell you a story:

I had a second practice in a neighboring town in Georgia, just across the state line. Once a month I performed a group channeling there. There was a woman who came nearly every time. She was always disruptive, seeking attention, talking behind my back, and actually sneering at me at times. I had a mild awareness of her, and I found her behavior to be very strange since I didn't even know her. In the interest of maintaining my balance and that of the group who had come to experience the Masters, I just brushed the whole thing off.

Never once did she speak to me directly during that time. She did come to one of the group meetings at my home and proceeded to challenge me at every turn. Each time she talked to me, she got right in my face, making a statement of her talents or gifts. Back then I was always excited to meet anyone who might have had even some of the experiences I had, so when she stated what she knew, what she could do, I was interested. I asked her specific questions, trying to determine the extent of her awareness.

I didn't do this to be judgmental at all. I did it looking for anyone who could comprehend some of the things that I had experienced. My world by then had gotten quite surreal, and I was still new at it all. It would have been great to be able to compare notes with someone else! Instead of her comparing notes with me, however, it was more like she wanted to pick a fight, and that was never anything that I was interested in. The whole thing was bizarre. She only showed up that once at my home but continued to appear at my monthly events, still being disruptive in the background.

Several years went by and I hadn't seen her. Then one day out of the blue, I received a call from her. The conversation went something like this:

"Hi, Meg. I would like to set up an appointment for a healing session with you."

A bit stunned to hear this, I asked her "Why *me?* I didn't get the impression that you respected my work very much."

"Well, I know that you are the only one who can help me, and I have avoided you for a long time because of that."

Okay . . . that was honest. I imagined that whatever her crisis was, it must have taken a lot of courage for her to call me. I had no idea what to expect, but I set an immediate appointment for her. I knew there was more to this picture than I had realized, but I had *no idea* the extent of what I was about to encounter!

Our appointment time came around, and as I always do with my clients, I sat and chatted with her, getting to know her a bit and directly asking her what it was she wanted me to help her with. She started explaining that none of the relationships in her life were working. She hadn't been able to hold a job, she had basically lost most of her friends, and life in general was going down the tubes. She was sincere in her desire to make a change and yet completely unaware as to why things were going the way they were.

After our conversation I took her into my healing room and proceeded to get to work. I was thinking that self-image or self-worth issues were contributing to her apparent failures in every direction of her life. Boy, was I wrong!

As I harmonized with her energy field, something felt off. There was too much energy, and it wasn't in focus. I can't quite explain the feeling, but it was almost as if her energy field had slid sideways.

I had been concentrating on the energy with my eyes closed, and when I opened them, I was startled as I looked down at my client. What I saw was far from being her. Instead, on my table lay a full-sized male reptilian being. Its scaled skin was gorgeous, reflecting light in an opalescent manner. It had thighs and muscles that felt like bricks, hard and dense. It emanated an inner strength that I hadn't encountered before. At the ends of his appendages were nails that looked more like short talons. They were kind of yellowish white, and they curved over the tips of the fingers and toes. Its shape was mostly humanoid, but it sure didn't feel that way.

In the same manner as my client, the reptilian being lay on the table peacefully with his eyes closed.

"Oh geeze. (Oh, yeah . . . keep breathing!) Uh Oh (God this is bizarre!). Now what?"

This was the first time I had seen anything like this and I needed to make sure that I did the right thing and didn't hurt my client or endanger myself at the same time.

My gut reflex was to separate this thing out of the poor woman, but at the same time, the Masters, my infinite guides who are always present, said an unequivocal "No! If you do that, you will kill her!"

"Oh . . . Kaaaaayyyyyy . . ."

Almost within the same breath I heard and thought, "Assimilate them."

"You have got to be kidding!" I thought. Meanwhile, while I am having this cosmic holy cow discussion, my client(s) rested peacefully on the table.

So I began assimilating the energies in the way I knew how. I closed my eyes and concentrated, commanding the energies to do what needed to be done. The two sets were vitally different from each other and my first attempt wasn't enough.

I looked down at one point, and what I saw was something out of a gory nightmare. My client looked like a human/reptilian version of the Philadelphia experiment. Stories about that event reveal a scientific experiment in electromagnetic forces going terribly wrong when the time-space continuum was interrupted by the powerful emissions of energy and the ship filled with navy men disappeared. When it returned, it was no longer a ship filled with men, but instead a combined mess of twisted metal and body parts.

What I saw looked like an entanglement of human and reptilian tissues and parts. There was no sense to any of it. Part of me was forever repulsed while another part of me was fascinated, and I kept working. I have to tell you at this point there were a lot of thoughts and feelings going through this girl. It was horrifying and curious all at the same time. It was at once gruesome and beautiful watching the forces of creation at work. I kept my wits about me, determined to complete what I had so timidly begun. God, who would ever believe this one! I guessed it didn't matter, because here we all were and I had to keep going. I admit that I was awed, shaken, and insatiably curious about the whole thing, but somehow I was never afraid.

I continued working with the harmonics of the two beings until they became fully assimilated and all that was visible in any world was the form of my client. A relief to speak mildly. I could still feel the energy of the reptilian, but it had assimilated into a powerful force within my human client. Her eyes actually changed shape and color. I was awed. And all this time she had no idea what was happening to her. Boy, this would be one for the records.

I always talk with my clients after the session as well as before, telling them what I found, what changes were made, and how they can do their part toward changing their experience further or maintaining the work we have done. This time I was at a loss for words. I mean, really, what do you tell someone in that kind of situation? The truth. I had to.

After a while, we went back out into the sitting area and I explained to her that I had some rather strange things to tell her. I tentatively began to describe what I had seen, what had been done, the whole thing. I half expected her to flee out the door, running for the hills. Instead she began to nod her head.

"This makes total sense! Now *so much* makes sense!"

Not at all what I had imagined she might say. I didn't know whether I should be relieved or what, so I just kept listening.

She proceeded to tell me that she had spent several years with a couple who were kind of surrogate parents to her. She told me she had somehow discovered that they were reptilians, and when she realized it, she had left immediately but that it had been a little too late. She went on to tell me of some of her experiences there, and none of them were good.

Not only was she hanging out with an enclave of reptilians, she had been playing with opening her consciousness and channeling whomever and whatever came through or into her body without any discernment or protection. By being so promiscuous with her self, she had unwittingly invited this creature into her body and life from that moment had been one challenging disaster after another.

She was so relieved after the session that she must have thanked me a million times. Her eye color had changed, as did her countenance and facial expressions. She was harmonized to nearly normal but with some side benefits. After that session, she went on to completely change her life. Things started going really well for her. Gone were the signs of aggression and passive–aggression. She found someone to have a good long–term relationship with and began to work as an animal communicator. Last I heard, she was becoming pretty well known for her good work with animals.

The other two types of reptilians are not pretty in any way. Maybe in some other world but certainly not ours. One type is dark green/brown and has a tail that trails the ground behind it. The tail is thick at its base and tapers off to a point at the end. These are the meanest, most destructive and aggressive of the reptilians. They are masters of deceit and are excellent shape shifters, propagating their lies by changing form to represent people we are comfortable with. When they reveal themselves, their red eyes can be frightening and haunt us for a long time after we see them.

The other kind of reptilian is often red or brown with a somewhat shorter tail that falls just below the knees. They have larger scales and seem to be an inter-dimensional creature that doesn't affect us too often. Both are extremely negative and emanate pure meanness and darkness.

Reptilians are opportunists who look for a human host to control for their personal agendas. They feed off the energy of human beings and are very alien harmonically.

Separation of reptilians from a human being's energy field is tricky. The longer they have been there, the more harmonized their energy fields become in relation to the human form. If they are caught early on before any real assimilation takes place, they can be removed and banished out of the human's field.

If they have been there a while and some assimilation has begun, they have to be assimilated with the human being. This kind of assimilation is a bit different because it requires harmonizing the energy of the human being to override the reptilian influences. Once done, the reptilian becomes an insignificant aspect of the human's energy field and harmless from that point on.

Entities

Entities are beings from lower dimensions that usually feed on negative energies and emotions. They can also cause them. Entities come in a variety of forms and intensities and are fairly common, affecting the unsuspecting. They can be present in our environment, waiting for someone to affect or to latch onto. Most entities are parasitic, stealing energy from their victims.

Entities are other-dimensional beings that have learned to closely harmonize with our energy fields. They are excellent at hiding within our Etheric anatomy and can be difficult to detect.

Early on, when I began working with the Etheric anatomy of my clients, after completing a full evaluation and attunement, I often felt as if something still wasn't quite right. It was as if there was an unseen, unidentifiable imbalance lurking just outside of my awareness. Upon changing my "sight" perspectives, I discovered that this particular set of feelings was correct. There were entities hiding within the energy fields, and they were pros at it!

Not all entities are scary or mean. Some are simple parasites that latch onto our energy fields, taking whatever they need from us. Others are downright nasty creatures who cause us all manner of problems, while still others can actually possess a person and turn even the meekest of people into rude, mean, uncaring specimens of humanity. Of course when that happens, it isn't the person at all, but the entity that is affecting them.

Entities can be picked up from other people too, like ticks and fleas; they are pests that we don't want. Most of us are not affected by entities, but we may at times be temporarily affected by them. If someone in our home has picked up one or more of the hitchhikers, we will feel it in their behavior and their attitudes.

The symptoms of entity attachment vary. Here is a list of mild to severe warning signs:

* Lack of focus or decisiveness

* Periods of great fatigue

* Unpredictable emotions; happy one minute, irate the next, for example

* Unexplained anger and negativity

* Mild to deep depression for no apparent reason

* Life isn't going well—there is a lot of chaos and negative experiences as well as failures even in simple situations.

* Argumentative

* Irrational and unreasonable behavior

* Self-destructive tendencies

* Addictive behaviors particularly with drugs and alcohol

* Suicidal thoughts and tendencies

* Abundance and lack issues

Of course the symptoms may vary in combination and intensity, but these are good guidelines.

When we are around someone who has one or more entities, we find that we are instinctively uncomfortable. There is an indescribable sense that something isn't quite right, but we can't seem to name what we are feeling. If a loved one has picked up an entity, we might find that their behavior is far from nice and there seems to be no explanation for it.

People who have entities aboard most often have no idea that this has happened to them. They don't understand why they suddenly feel the way they do and become very defensive when asked about it.

To a practitioner, the energy of an entity will feel at once heavy and sharp and as if it is in front of them, separate from the client's energy field. This is a very subtle feeling but obvious once we have tuned into it.

There are several types of entities that I have encountered over the years:

Nesters

Nesters are other-dimensional entities that have been inserted into our energy fields. They are almost always in multiples and are curled up in the abdominal cavity. I have seen nesters in an energy field that have been there for an indeterminate amount of time. I have the sense that the entities have been attached to the energy field long before the current lifetime of the client.

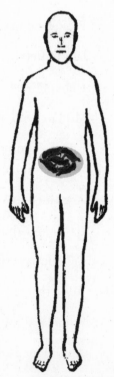

Nesters are fairly harmless. In their multiple occupation, all curled up together in the abdominal area, they remind me of a barely vital litter of puppies. In their cozy place they seem to be incubating. They are about six inches long. They have very little vitality, almost as if they are in a state of suspended animation, but still they are drawing vital energy from the host's system. Nesters mostly cause lack of clarity and focus and fluctuating emotional, physical, and mental energies. They can affect the physical body, causing digestive and reproductive issues or low back pain.

Nesters hide in the abdomen.

Removing nesters is not difficult. They are simply lifted out of the system, then transmuted to either light energy or inert matter. Sometimes they have formed a dense shell around their area that is really dense energy but is fragile and can shatter like an eggshell. This is part of their camouflage. As soon as we access the gestating entities, we break the protective shell. Care must be taken to search for and alleviate all pieces of this wall because if something is missed, it can cause inflammation in the energy field and later physical illness such as abscess or organ issues as well as cysts or tumors.

Symbiotic Parasitic Entities

There is another kind of entity that causes some of the more serious problems in our list. These are entirely parasitic. This type of entity can be about four feet in length. They latch onto the energy field by sinking their long hooked teeth into the mid-back or heart area. Usually, they latch on in the mid-back.

People who are carrying these kinds of entities will change behavior and even their clothing styles to reflect how they feel. For example, I was at an expo, running a booth to sell my books, and I felt a dark negative presence in the crowd. As my eyes scanned the crowd to find what I felt, they landed on a tall, good-looking dark-haired young man of late high school age. He was dressed in an extremely gothic manner with black lipstick and fingernails, and he was carrying a pack with him that had all sorts of underworld symbols on it. He was literally hunched partially over, and I wondered why.

As he neared me, I saw that he had an entity attached to his back that was one of the largest of this type I had seen. Its teeth were hooked into the spinal area of the young fellow's mid-back. Often when entities attach, they affect the posture of

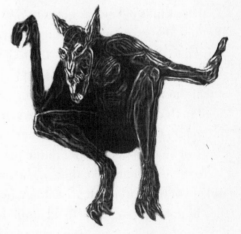

The Symbiotic Parasitic Entity latches onto the mid-back and influences the behavior of its victim in order to create more negative emotions and energy to feed on.

the person because they are an energetic weight and their attachment causes the energy system to have to compromise its flow patterns in order to adapt to the intruder.

The young man's behavior was mimicking the energy of the dark being who was both stealing his life force and instigating further destructive behavior in order to generate more negative energy to feed on. The more the young man personified and acted upon the energies of the entity, the more powerful the entity had become. Without realizing it, this young man had become a symbiotic vessel for the entity's persona and activities.

I watched as he walked by, transfixed at what I was witnessing. That this fellow and his attachment showed up at that expo fascinated me. The entire expo was filled with light workers and the speakers were of high caliber and definite purveyors of light.

These kinds of entities are drawn to light workers like moths to flame, but they cannot access the light at all. When they realize this, they become troublemakers. As he went by, I noticed that he had attracted other, less strong people who had begun to follow him. Some of them had entities attached to them as well, but nothing to the strength or degree that the young man had.

These kinds of entities may often be very resistant when we try to remove them. They are also excellent at hiding within the energy field and can, believe it or not, be hard to identify as separate from the energy field of a person. Quite often, if I suspect entity attachment and I am working long distance, I will set a time for the appointment and then do the session the night before or way later than I had indicated so that I can access the entities unannounced. If they know we are accessing the energy field, they hide like Etheric chameleons. When they are unsuspecting, they can be very easy to spot immediately upon access of the client's Etheric field.

To remove them, take them tightly by the scruff of the neck and lift them up and out of their attached area. Then, hold them up into the light and demand that they be gone. As we make that command, the entities de-particulate and turn into particulates of light, waiting to be re-created as some other part or aspect of creation that is no longer of darkness. It is important to remember to repair the area where the entity was attached since it would have puncture wounds in the energy field as well as inflammation and often areas of density or stagnant energy. This can be done by commanding that the area normalize and then attune.

Hitchhikers

Hitchhikers are temporary entities that are literally hitching a ride with their victims. Usually, the victim isn't aware that anything unworldly is going on. They are more of a nuisance than anything but can mildly to moderately affect their victims in a variety of ways.

Hitchhikers don't actually attach to the victim like some of the other entities. Instead, they glom onto the energy field and use it to feed their own energy system until they get where they are going.

The victim is usually unaware of the hitchhiker's presence and goes about his business oblivious to the fact that he is being used as a transportation vehicle for otherworldly beings from the darker realities.

Hitchhikers seem to travel in packs of several or more and are often prevalent in certain geographical areas, particularly where there have been battles fought or periods of extreme violence. For example, the Atlanta area saw much violence during the Civil War. There were prison camps and hospitals, hidden assets such as gold of the Confederacy, and a great deal of fighting. Healers in that area report an uncommon number of hitchhikers there. Southern California is another area where there are a lot of these pests. There were times during the Spanish occupation that slaves were used and bloody battles were fought over territories. Hitchhikers are certainly not limited to these areas and can be found pretty much anywhere.

The hitchhikers will hop off in different locations when they feel that they have either reached their destination or when they find an area that is suitable to their energy needs.

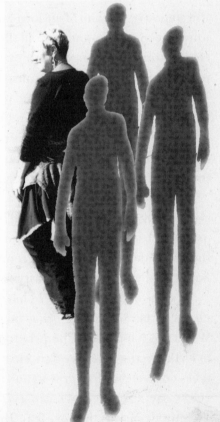

Most of us don't realize we have hitchhikers.

Years ago, I worked with a fifteen-year-old girl from the Atlanta area. She had gotten heavily involved with the dark side of witchcraft and was running a very destructive coven in underground Atlanta. When she came in, I could feel the entities all over her. As I worked on her, I found several different types of them and destroyed them. Later, after she and her mother left, I went into my living room where we had originally met and talked. There were hitchhikers everywhere, nearly twenty of them. Knowing that I would be working on her and removing any darkness-related affectations, they had basically jumped ship and landed in my living room. Ugh! A lot of light, some good clearing, and a few serious commands got them out of there!

Possession and Infestation by Groups of Entities

Infestation by a group of entities can be a terrible experience. Entities gather like unruly teenagers in and around the field of the victim and change its frequencies to more closely match their own. Their presence can cause all manner of problems in a person's life because their energy is extremely dark and negative. They are particularly attracted to people who habitually take recreational drugs, particularly the stronger ones and hallucinogens, or drink heavily. These types of entities love it when a person is not in control of her faculties and they can take over. When they do, often they cause serious behavioral anomalies in their victims and they propagate self-destructive behavior as well.

This kind of entity affectation is one of the worst because the group members are actually just flunkies for a much worse kind of entity. Most of the time, when a group such as this is present, there is one very vicious controlling entity running the entire show from the background. The individuals in the group are merely puppets for the desires of a nasty demonic creature.

In some of the worst cases I have seen, members of the group possess their victim for periods of time. They take over the body and mind of their victim. When this happens, the body becomes very sick and has a particularly vile odor to it. The victim will have dark rings under his eyes and foul breath. The skin takes on a yellowish or gray pallor, and often the victim will speak in altered voices, saying crude and mean-spirited things to anyone who interferes.

Entities such as this love fear. They love decadence and will cause the victim to engage in behaviors that she would never otherwise do, such as promiscuous sex acts, alteration by more drugs and alcohol, violent acts, and even self-destructive acts such as cutting the body, even suicide at times.

The only way to rid a victim of these kinds of entities is to destroy the one who is running them in the background, and it isn't an easy task. I will talk more about this in a moment.

The worst kind of entity involvement occurs when an entity, usually a demonic type, possesses the body of the victim. When the dark force becomes present in the body, it is strengthened by the life force of the victim. There is literally nothing that a victim of possession won't do, because it isn't the victim in action but, rather, the entity and its crude and vile desires. Telling you a story that is at once disturbing yet true will best help to describe this situation.

We had recently moved to a new state over three thousand miles from my home of twenty years. I didn't know anyone and was feeling a bit lost. I found a little metaphysical store in town and went in, hoping to learn about like-minded people and activities in the area. I had visited the store two or three times and found really nothing of value to my desires. I was looking around at some new book arrivals when I heard the proprietor say, "Ask Meg. I bet she will know."

"Hmm," I thought, "I wonder what is up."

The store owner introduced me to a pleasant young woman who was fairly cheerful but was also overweight and didn't look particularly healthy. When I looked at her I had a nebulous sense that something was very wrong. The young woman told me that for eight years there had been presences in her house that were unexplained and that often caused problems. She told me that objects often flew across the room and other bizarre things happened. She said it was strange because the kinds of spirits that came and went changed nearly every month. Sometimes they seemed harmless, while at other times they were not so good. Her attitude was kind of devil-may-care about the whole thing. She even said at one point that she had become used to "them" because "they" had been there so long, but she knew they really had to go. She wondered if I could come and "clear" her house.

Easy enough, I thought. Most likely an open portal that is allowing crossovers of spirits from different levels of dimensions.

"Sure, I can come over and see what we can do to help you out."

Not exactly the kind of spiritual connections I had been looking for, but I did know a lot about this subject, or so I thought.

On our agreed day and time I went to her home. When I walked in the front door, I immediately was hit with a wall of dark and disturbing energy. As I looked around, there were pentagrams and other symbols and indications of witch-craft everywhere. Mostly books and innocuous objects, but I made a mental note because sometimes when people practice witchcraft and begin to dabble in the dark arts, they open doors to darkness that are only the beginning of nightmar-ish experiences. I have nothing against witchcraft, by the way, when it is prac-ticed in the light. It is when that line is crossed into the dark side and forces are unleashed that can become intractable that I become very concerned.

As I crossed the threshold into the house, the young woman told me that she wanted me to meet her son. He was four years old. I hadn't noticed him before that moment because the energy in the house was so negative and I was focused on that.

She scooped up her son in her arms and swung back around to me.

"Meet my son, Billy!" (not his real name).

I love kids. As many know, I advocate for the Children of Now in every way and was doing so at that time as well. As she swung around, I moved closer to greet the little guy, but what I saw, heard, and smelled made me reel with disgust.

The little four-year-old smelled so vile that it was literally nauseating. I imme-diately knew the meaning of the smell of brimstone. His teeth were rotten, his skin nearly transparent. He was way too thin, and just short of emaciated. Uncondi-tionally, I reached up to touch him and . . . he reeled back, leaning away from me.

"GET OUT OF HERE!" he said in a very adult male growl. I can't tell you how shocking and disturbing it was to witness this coming from a little guy. This was like the movie, *The Exorcist*, but his head didn't spin. It might as well have.

"Oh, Jesus." I spoke to myself, "I know what this is. I can't be afraid. Angels protect me; this isn't a house clearing; this little boy is possessed!"

And with every ounce of righteous indignation I could muster, I said right back into his face, "I am not leaving. YOU ARE!"

It spoke back to me in a language I can only describe as being from hell itself. Its message was vile and livid. It wanted me gone.

The young mom laughed and said, "Isn't he cute? He has been talking in voices like that practically since he was born. He has so many invisible friends!"

I knew from experience that dark entities couldn't take the touch of some-one who works with the light. It is like acid to them. I can't tell you how many thoughts went through my mind in a split second. My mind was reeling, as were every one of my senses. What had I gotten into? What do I do now? It went something like this:

(Several expletives that I won't repeat here) then:

"My God this poor child!"

"Is she that ignorant that she can't see that her son isn't normal? That he is possessed by something awful? Surely not?"

"I don't know this woman, and I just told her son he is leaving."

"Oh, God, what have I gotten myself into?"

"I can't be afraid no matter what."

"Okay. Buck up here, don't back down for any reason."

"I need to use every protection I can."

I inquired about Billy's health because I was greatly concerned about him. His mom laughed and said he didn't eat much and that he never slept through the night. In fact, none of his habits were very normal, but isn't he cute? And then I politely turned back to the mom and asked to be shown the entire house.

My tour of the home led me from the living room to the boy's bedroom. It was a wreck as if someone had gone wild and thrown everything into disarray. We moved through the upstairs somewhat uneventfully. Then we proceeded downstairs to the basement.

With each step I took downward, the energy became worse. It went from dark to foreboding. I could feel violence and mayhem. The first room I saw when we got to the bottom of the stairs looked like a bomb had exploded. It was meant for storage, but there was no order and tons of trash strewn everywhere.

I looked through an adjoining doorway to a room that looked much more pleasant . . . until I got closer and saw the aquarium. It held a rather large boa constrictor. Serpents. Great.

"Oh, that is Billy's pet!" Mom said.

How appropriate, a four-year-old with a snake that could choke him out at any minute.

"Usually, we let him run loose when Billy is playing down here," Mom said.

I asked her to leave the snake in its cage.

And then I looked up. There was a closed door across the room and on it was a poster of a skeleton in female bordello type attire splayed out in a promiscuous pose. I can't describe it more than to say its leering grin was over the top. Under the circumstances, it wasn't funny.

"What's behind this door?" I needed to know. I was feeling that the focus area of darkness was in there. In fact, I was feeling a powerful portal. We were below ground level at this point.

"It's my husband's ammunition room. He makes his own ammunition and also makes knives."

Elements of death. Yes, well . . .

And then the door was opened for me. A rush of dank air escaped from the room. This was the heart of the dark forces in the house. It was originating right here. On the workbench was a mirror with yet another skeleton. There were tools and weapons in various stages in there. Bullets, knives, the works. The room was all concrete, like a vault.

Separately, none of these signs would have been particularly worrisome, but their combination and the number of them was a clear sign that dark forces were at work in that house.

With my inner sight, I saw that a portal was open. It was huge and forceful, but there was something odd about it. I wasn't sure what. Honestly, I was winging it at the time. I had never seen such a combination of dark energies and weirdness in my life. At the same time, I was at once terrified and fascinated.

This was without a doubt the place to start. I asked the family to leave me alone down there so that I could "get into my space" and assess what was going on. I told them I might be a while. They left me there and sent the little guy to a neighbor to be watched.

I sat on a stool in the room and quickly accessed multiple dimensions. I saw that the portal was accessing multiple realities in a cyclic manner. Portals are like apertures that may often open and close rhythmically. As creation pulses, it moves, and the alignments of portals may or may not align into another reality. What was unique about this one was that it was opening and closing in and out of dimensional realities in a predictable cycle. This was why the young woman experienced different kinds of spirits in her home regularly. Some of the doorways the portal accessed were simply to the spirit world. I witnessed the spirits of departed souls coming and going. Most of them were from the nineteenth century.

Pioneers who had come from the east along the Oregon Trail had settled the area there. The spirits were dressed in pioneer fashion, the men in breeches and the women in puffy dresses and wearing bonnets. There was a feel of innocence about them, but also a sense of disturbed earnest. They moved about as if they didn't know where to go but did so with great purpose as if maybe a turn to the left or the right might finally take them where they wanted to go.

There were other spirits too. They were from different times and places. The portal here allowed a who's who of beings from different times and realities to come and go. Unfortunately, as it changed planes of access, those who had come through the doorway had become trapped. The entities had also found the doorway long ago when the portal had entered into their dimensional doorways, and they had taken full advantage of it, living off the energy of this family and likely others before them.

I had closed portals before so had a sense of what to do here, but this one was different because of its multiple accesses. In order to keep the spirits and others from being forever trapped on the wrong side of the portal, I had to send them all back to their various realities. I sent out a telepathic call to all of those who had crossed into the area. I called them to return home. I had no idea what to expect and what I witnessed was nothing short of amazing. As I controlled the aperture of the portal, souls who had been trapped there for centuries began to line up to go home. There were hundreds of them. They were from varying periods in time and all forms of life. It was bizarre. If I hadn't been watching it with my own eyes, I would have sworn I had made it all up. I couldn't have. I hadn't. When I looked back over my shoulder I saw that they stood in line to enter back through the portal as far as I could see.

There were a few stragglers who I had to find before closing the portal. As they came, I encouraged them to cross back over through their respective dimensional doorways. For the most part, they were quite relieved to find their way back until I encountered a nasty group of dark beings. All of the rest of the beings had gone to their respective levels of reality, but these guys weren't going to budge. A stubborn lot, their intentions were nothing good, and they felt vicious and destructive. Okay, here it comes.

I knew that in order to relieve this home and its occupants of its horrible situation, I had to destroy these creatures and their source. These things weren't just in the wrong neighborhood; they had effectively achieved a coup that included not only the house but also nearly everyone in it.

I diligently went about attempting to destroy the pests. Usually, pesky entities can be banished and will go away when commanded. This wasn't the case here. I had to destroy them in order for the little boy to survive.

Oddly, the more I destroyed, the more there were. It seemed like there was an endless army of demonic beings who were determined to maintain their hold on the place. After a short time, I realized that I was getting nowhere. I decided to look for their source. By now, I had begun to suspect a secondary portal or something, but what I found was far from that.

Ethereally I waded through the pesky entities, looking for a way to stop them. As my consciousness went through from one dimension to another, I came to a place that felt so empty it was as if a vacuum had sucked all of the energy out of it. As I looked around, I felt an evil so vile that there are no words to describe it. I looked up, and there stood a demon of the nastiest caliber I could have imagined. He was the embodiment of everything depraved and loathsome. He looked it, and he felt like it. I knew at once that he was the source of all the flunkies. He was sending them to do his malevolent bidding and reaping the benefits of his army's work. He was sucking the energy from his flunkies as they robbed the household and the family of theirs. I realized that every member of the group was expendable, and there were plenty more where they came from, but this one was much different.

As soon as I laid eyes in him, I knew that he was the one who actually possessed the little boy. He was malicious and evil to the core. He reeked of the same smell I had sensed in the boy, and he oozed a putrid scum around his mouth. His teeth were ragged and he emanated everything terrible. He snarled at me, and I knew that this encounter was going to come down to him or me. It became a moment of survival. One of us would die right there and right then. There was no turning back because not only had I discovered him, he had seen me.

Without thinking, I reached over my shoulder to my back and grabbed my light sword. I had discovered it years earlier but had no idea what it was for. I was about to find out. I held the sword into the light above me, and it seemed to energize. There were arcs of light, like cosmic lightning, striking the blade. As they did, the blade began to glow brightly. It was so bright it hurt my ethereal eyes.

I thrust my light sword into the beast, and when it impaled his heart, the beast exploded into countless pieces. There was a sound like thunder that filled the vacuum space and then silence followed by a sense of peace. I was breathing hard from the intensity of the moment, and as my breath slowed back to normal, I was impressed by how still the house felt. It felt empty. They were gone.

I sat there for a bit and recovered my senses. This experience was a far stretch of altered reality into realms of darkness that were far beyond my usual scope. I was having trouble even believing what had just happened, but I knew it was real, and knowing that made it somehow even worse.

I checked my energy field thoroughly for any entities that may have latched on and found it clear of any problems. I took a little more time to collect myself and tried to decide just what to say to these people who I had just met. I decided to play it by ear and see how things went when I went upstairs.

When I went back to the main floor, I was reeling from the experience. I was worried about the little guy. I didn't see him anywhere. His parents told me that he was still at the neighbor's. I asked to see him immediately.

When the neighbor brought the little boy home, I was stunned at what I saw. Little Billy had lost the darkness under his eyes. He was laughing and play-ing. His skin tone had changed to a more normal, healthy looking flesh, and his energy field no longer had the dense, vile aspects it had earlier. The horrific smell was gone too.

I explained to the parents that there had been a portal with some pretty awful things coming and going and left it at that for the time being because I didn't know them well enough to go into the details of hell. They were very grateful, to say the least. I still had a nagging feeling that the whole thing wasn't over yet, but I revisited the experience in my head over and over and couldn't find anything left undone. I was focused on the boy and the house.

I stayed for a while, watching the boy with deep gratitude as his complexion and every other aspect of him normalized. Before I left, he came and threw his arms around me and said, "I love you, Meg!" That was the greatest hug I ever had in my life. That he could do that told me there were no remnants of evil left in his little being.

His mom called me the next day and said that Billy was eating like a horse and that he had slept all night. She couldn't believe the difference in him. I was so happy to know that he would now survive and grow to be a normal child who was filled with joy rather than the alternative he had faced before.

Since we had just moved to the area, we hadn't found a permanent place to live yet, and we were staying in a local motel. That night I went to sleep, exhausted from the amount of energy that I had used that day. Later in the night, I was awakened by a loud male voice that growled, *"Who are you?!"*

The voice was similar to the one that had spoken to me through the boy. Oh, geeze, something has followed me home! And then I got mad. Really mad. They had *no right* to bother me!

I stated my name. I said that I was of the light, with the light, and within the light. I demanded that it be gone. It left. And it never came back to me or to my new little four-year-old friend again.

I was so profoundly affected by the whole experience that I visited the family regularly for several years, keeping an eye on the little guy. He began to grow normally and took an interest in horseback riding, fishing, and boating with his dad. His mother, oddly, wouldn't let me too close to her for the first couple of years. I noticed that her health was declining in multiple ways. Her weight gain worsened, her eyes began to weep constantly, and she began having female problems and several other undiagnosed issues. She wouldn't let me work on her. Period. Ultimately, I worked on half of the neighborhood as other homes and people had been affected by the infestation of nastiness that had been there. There was a lot of cleaning up to do. Mom was the only one I hadn't worked on. Finally, one day she called.

"I miss them," she said. "It is so quiet around here. I was so used to hearing their voices that I just about can't stand the silence. I feel so alone."

"In your case, silence is a very good thing," I said laughingly.

"I know, but still . . . anyway, I was thinking . . . I think I am ready for you to work on me now."

This was about two years after I had cleared the house and Billy of the infestation.

"Sure, happy to."

We set an appointment and I went over there. She was kind of apprehensive but had gotten so sick she was getting desperate for some help. As I accessed her field, I realized that she was carrying multiple entity attachments. They were the reason for her illnesses. They writhed around her abdominal area in an attempt to hide from me and in that moment I had a revelation.

Billy had become possessed in utero. As he grew in her belly, the entities began to possess him. This was why the mother never realized that something was wrong with him. He had always been that way, and there had been no moment in time, no drastic change in him for her to see a difference.

It was the mom who had practiced the dark arts. Mostly out of ignorance. She hadn't meant any harm. She honestly didn't know the difference. The entities had attached to her so cloaked in deception that she never even realized they were there until I ran them off, away from her home. Those that were left had attached into her energy field and needed to be addressed directly.

I was able to remove them, and she began to be healthy again. For a while at least. Later she began to be sick again but did not ask for my help.

About four years later, I was presenting at an expo in the area and as I looked up, I saw this family approaching me. Billy had grown into a stocky young guy, healthy and happy. He wanted to show me how he had learned to meditate. He sat cross-legged in front of me, put his hands together and zoned right out, oblivious to the crowds there. He sat there for the longest time and then finally popped back in. His parents were so proud of him. I was too, and I advised them to make sure that he knows safety rules about traveling with his consciousness. He had been through enough already, but I felt he would be okay. For years Billy's parents sent me pictures of him in his various childhood activities. What a blessing to know that this soul was pulled from the mouths of hell. I have wondered over the years just what he will do with his life. Time will tell.

The story of Billy and his family is unusual in the sense that it encompassed so many different attributes and types of spirits and beings. My greatest sense was that the entity occupation was of such long standing and strength in the energy it had built up, it attracted other entities and opened doors to further realms of reality as its arachnid hold on the house and its inhabitants intensified.

Later, as I examined the grounds around the house, I found that two men had died in a conflict and bled into the ground right above the weapons room of the basement. There was a lot of intense emotional charge imprinted in the area that likely attracted the entities in the first place. Fear, war, and even bloody death, were all contributive to setting up energies there for a portal to open and a hellish feast as the entities gathered there. But not anymore.

Portals

There are different types of portals. Most of them serve to maintain balance between dimensions. Some of them are accessible to us while some are not. One type of portal really isn't a portal at all but can be classified as such. This type is called a vortex. We have different vortexes in our Etheric anatomy, such as our chakras and the yin and yang vortexes that we talked about earlier.

There is another type of vortex that comes up from the earth and its magnetic field. These range in size and intensity, and when we stand in them we may be able to access other dimensions for a short time. These kinds of portals can be positive or negative in polarity and spin and are often found on *ley lines*, or parts of the earth's energy grid system. Vortexes can be male or female, and there are usually signs in the immediate area indicating their presence. Earth vortexes almost always have at least one guardian tree, and sometimes as many as three. These trees are generally very old and large. When there are three, they are usually spaced around the vortex in an equilateral triangular shape. There may also be a circular area on the ground where either nothing grows at all or different types of growth unusual for that particular area may be found.

Sometimes there are double or triple vortexes. When this occurs they are usually of alternating polarities. In other words, two are usually male and female, positive and negative polarities, and triples are usually alternating polarities such as positive, negative, positive. There are exceptions to this rule, but these are most common.

The next type of portal is the dimensional portal, much like what I dealt with in the story of Billy. Dimensional portals are not usually stationary, and they open and close in the natural rhythm of creation. These kinds of portals can become stuck in an open or closed position. They can be accessed by our consciousness and in rare instances by our entire beings, including our bodies.

Some dimensional portals allow access to more than one reality over time. As creation pulses and moves rhythmically, the portal crosses the apertures to several different dimensions and allows access on both sides of the gateway. Other portals only access one reality in addition to ours. These openings in the fabric of creation maintain balance and pressure among dimensions.

A third type of portal was created eons ago for a specific purpose. These act as doorways into and out of multi-dimensional wormhole systems. They can be entered and exited only by those who are able to reach certain levels of consciousness. These portals are much like the vacuum systems that many bank drive-throughs have. When we enter them, we are sucked into them at an indescribable pace. Then, once we reach certain heights in these portals, there are hubs where we can change direction. These hubs often look like wheels with spokes, having multiple turn offs accessible that are at specific angulations. There are portals like this in many places on Earth such as in some of the underground temples in Egypt and the Doorway of Lord Aramu Muru in Peru.

Lord Aramu Muru is said to have come through the portal from another world, bringing the solar disk, a solid gold artifact that became the most sacred object of worship in all of the Incan lands. The disk hung prominently on a high exterior wall of the Qorikancha, the temple of the sun. Legend has it that when word of the Conquistador's impending raid came, the disk was whisked away and hidden under the waters of Lake Titicaca. These powerful doorways to other parts of the multiverse, when in open mode, have been known to suck people in so that they never return.

There is a story about the doorway of Lord Aramu Muru in which four wandering musicians were crossing the nearby fields. One of them was tired and lagged behind while the other three kept walking up into the rock hills. The fourth musician eventually caught up to where his compadres had gone but they were nowhere to be found. He could hear them playing music far in the distance, but they and everything they carried had vanished from our world.

Stories abound even today amongst the villagers about the otherworldly musicians that can be heard playing in the hills from time to time.

These powerful portals were once used to travel instantly from one world to another, particularly in ancient Egypt, and have been referred to in ancient texts as doorways to the afterlife and doorways into the underworlds. It is through these doorways that those who were considered gods in pre-ancient Egypt times traveled in order to teach the ancient technologies to the Egyptians.

Visions of Cups and Swords, Rods and Disks

When I first began working in the Etheric worlds with clients, I began to encounter certain symbolic items in their energy fields. I saw chalices, usually by the throat, in people who were in the midst of or about to have immense spiritual awakenings. I found swords impaled in areas of chronic or acute pain. I found rods of various lengths and colors, and disks in various locations of the bodies. Often more than one kind of symbol was found. The swords and rods were generally found in angles of fifteen or more degrees. The disks were also usually angulated, and I considered them to be implants of some sort. I began to wonder if these symbolic shapes had something to do with past life experiences.

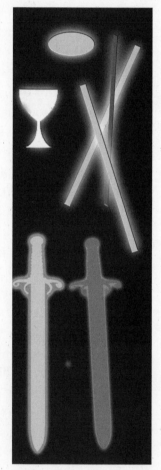

One day, one of my regular clients was in for a session. I found an unusual amount of these items in his field. There were three swords, a couple of rods, and something else. I told him that I really didn't understand the meaning of them except to say that when I pulled them out of the body, pain diminished or was altogether alleviated.

As a retired rocket scientist, my client was curious and did some research. On a whim, he got out his tarot book and looked up the respective numbers of the objects I had found. He called me later, very excited, to tell me that the objects I had found in his body exactly correlated with tarot cards of the same objects and numbers! Whatever the card descriptions had been fit his life to a tee. I came to realize that the tarot deck was most likely developed by someone who could see in the same otherworldly way that I did. It was a fun revelation to say the least.

Various items that are found in the Tarot may also occasionally be found in the Etheric field.

I noticed that when I found swords they were often presented in different ways in conjunction with the bodies of my clients. I also realized that there was more than one kind. When the swords were literally sticking through the body somewhere, there was physical pain. They would also be laid on top of the body point up (warrior presentation) or point down (peaceful presentation). I would also see them as two swords crossed in an X formation, which signified a compadre of someone.

I began to notice that there was more than one kind. There were metallic swords that varied in length and style, and there were swords of light of varying intensity. I came to learn that the metallic swords related to people who are spiritual warriors. The light swords were always found with healers. Not everyone has them, but those who do are intense in some aspects of their lives.

Some people carry both types,. as often a healer has to also be a warrior depending upon the kind of healing they are doing. It was the sword of light that I had unconsciously pulled in order to battle the demon that possessed Billy. I realized later that the swords come with those who are or have belonged to the Legions of Michael the Archangel. Often when the swords are pulled out, Michael will come and cleanse them before they are put away, or in cases like what happened with the demons, he will charge the swords with angelic light before they are used. The light swords can also be used for healing when all else fails.

Michael will also come and cleanse a sword after it is pulled from a body. Once the sword is cleansed, it should not be destroyed or discarded, but instead, laid on top of the body point down.

I know that this whole thing sounds like a very interesting make believe tale, but these swords and their uses are very real. At one point, I ran across several healers who didn't know each other and were finding similar swords with their clients. All of us got together and talked via email and put the pieces together.

The finding of swords, chalices, and rods also seems to come in phases. Perhaps none will be found for several years, and then it seems like a ton of people have them. The rods seem to be the most common and can be found more often than the other Tarot symbols.

ET Influences and Abductions

There is nothing more terrifying than awakening to hear a vibrating hum that moves through our bodies, affecting us to our very core. Simultaneously, the lights and electronics in the house may begin to flash off and on, and the air turns blue. As we resist, we might even hear a message in our head to, "Be still; it will be over quicker."

We believe we are in a dream, and in it various things are done to us, physical exams with probes or perhaps teachings with walls of living pictures that show us the future of our world. We dream of flying up through a shaft of light, through walls or windows, or falling back to our beds.

When we come back to our senses, we may be partially clothed or wearing no clothing at all, and we are not in the last position that we remember. But we can't remember anything except maybe the blue light or the hum, if that.

As we get dressed, we might notice that we have bruises on our bodies that we don't remember getting. We might have strange scars that are nearly healed that are little straight lines, V shapes, or little scoops out of our skin. These are curious, but we have no idea how we got them.

We might feel anxious or confused and not know why. We might begin to know things that are beyond our scope of experience or studies. We become afraid of closed places and the dark. Especially the dark. We don't want to be alone, but we need to be alone. We feel like we are being watched much of the time.

We have strange illnesses that the doctor can't name or figure out. We might run high fevers for no apparent reason, or suffer from temporary paralysis as a child or teenager. If we are female, we may have moderate to extreme problems with our reproductive systems, missed periods, endometriosis, or extreme menstrual bleeding. In some cases, we might be pregnant one day and not the next.

Or we may have no symptoms at all.

We may have no memories about these times at all.

But we can know that we are likely alien abductees.

These thoughts are frightening, but these kinds of examples happen to people every day. How many experience them is unknown because most are not reported, and many simply have no idea that this is happening to them.

Most often when someone is an abductee, he doesn't realize it but he has emotional and psychological, as well as physical, problems that he can't explain and can't seem to overcome. He may feel victimized, knowing that whatever is happening to him could happen again at any time, and he has no power to stop it. He wants to disconnect from the situation but doesn't know how. Sometimes he seeks alternative healing when all else fails him.

The alien abductee can have an odd assortment of unrelated complaints or concerns. Or she may just feel out of sorts, and sometimes these feelings are cyclical for no apparent reason.

On the flip side, many abductees are oblivious to anything out of the ordinary and come to the practitioner for other reasons.

Chances are that if someone has been abducted once, she has been abducted multiple times, some throughout their entire lives. It is also likely that others in the family have also been abducted.

There are many schools of thought on the whole alien abduction subject. Many will argue that it is a figment of very active imaginations, while others arduously argue that the phenomenon is very real. The truth is that too many people all over the planet over too many years share the same or similar stories. None of them have known each other or anything about the subject of UFOs, aliens, or alien abduction, but their stories are so similar and often identical in detail, experiences, remnant sensory experiences, and even gained intuitive or psychic abilities.

As a practitioner, over the years I have discovered quite a few abductees in various ways. Occasionally, those who have been abducted have implants inserted in their bodies that have harmonized with the system of the client, but they also have certain harmonics of their own that are outside of the scope of human energy systems. The difference is very subtle, but to an experienced practitioner, easy to find. We don't need to go looking for them, so to speak, on everyone we treat; usually if they are there, they will show up.

If we do know someone is an abductee, it is a good idea to scan their bodies for implants. When we are merged with the energy field, it is easy to move through the system methodically looking for anomalies.

We might also recognize an abductee by changes in their harmonics. The energy system of an abductee is different in resonance from what we usually see. The harmonics feel like a high-pitched sound does in our body. It is as if someone has turned up the gain and we have gotten our microphone too close to the speakers, creating a high-pitched squeal. Being with an abductee can feel like that, only the squeal is a lot higher frequency.

The reason the client's harmonics have changed so drastically is that when he is abducted, the vibrational hum that was described earlier shakes apart the particulates of the body, as well as the energy fields, so that it can be transported across the barriers of time and space. When a body de-particulates, it is a lot like what we used to see in Star Trek when Scotty beamed everyone up, only these trips are involuntary and there are some variances to the process. When the body re-assimilates, there are slight errors in the particulate arrangement. The errors do not usually cause harm but do cause the high frequency issues.

If we are sighted, seeing across the veils and into other levels of reality, when we work on an abductee, we might notice that we have company in the room with us. Extraterrestrials are very curious about any practitioner who is able not only to detect these anomalies, but also disengage them or re-harmonized them back to normal. They will come ethereally, stand in the room, and observe without interfering. Their curiosity overrules their need to control the situation.

Again, treating abductees is not for an inexperienced practitioner. It is a delicate process that requires a high command of energy and its nuances. A practitioner who does not completely understand these issues can do more damage than good.

Most of the people who are abducted are not aware of it. They just have a mixed bag of symptoms that they want help in dealing with. Sometimes the client will have some awareness and say something, or at least express their suspicions, but likely not.

I find that in dealing with abductees much discretion is advised. There is the dilemma of how much to say if someone is unaware. Tipping someone's reality that far can be their undoing. It can throw them into a crisis or a state of fear that is unbearable. Each case is individual in how it should be handled by the practitioner. How much we say depends upon the client, their openness and ability to consider expanded forms of reality. There have been times when I have candidly discussed the issue and others when I simply have made the required changes in the energy system and not gone into any detail about what I had found and changed.

Often we don't know our clients well enough to make that determination, and we can't let our own emotions or opinions rule in those situations. We must remain as responsible caregivers. Some would argue that we should tell every little detail about what we find. If a client had no awareness, sometimes not bringing that awareness forward is the biggest gift we can give them; when brought to the surface the memories and the experiences might be too much to handle, especially if they come crashing in because we opened the door.

On the other hand, if a client asks, or has some sort of awareness, it is a good idea to validate them. How much detail we give them again is relative to their openness and ability to consider all things strange. Some people will take their abduction experiences in stride while others will completely freak out.

In either case, whatever we find, we can change, correct, or, in the case of implants, disarm. The best thing to do is to bring the energy system and all of its levels back into normal balance. This is done in the same way we work on anyone else.

In the case of implants, there are many reasons they may be in place. Some gather data about the biology and the energy system of the client while others are tracking devices that make them easy to locate. Others regulate the energy system. These often give off real heat.

Examples of these are the ones that are often found in the cartilage of the ears. The ear will begin to emit a lot of heat, as if someone is rapidly turning up the thermostat. Later, the ear will itch to beat the band and nothing makes that itch stop. Yet others seem to bring information to their unsuspicious wearer, assisting them in knowing things about virtually any subject that they would have otherwise never known about.

All implants do not need to be disarmed, as some of them are actually assisting the client. Those that are tracking devices really should be eliminated. Once a practitioner has had several experiences with the different types of implants, believe it or not, he can tell the difference.

Implants come in various types, as we have discussed earlier. They can be forms of energy or hard copies and can be found virtually throughout the body but are usually in predictable places. Physically removing them can be impossible without drastically disfiguring a person, since they often morph to join the tissues so succinctly that they can't be separated out. Or, they simply migrate to a different area.

We can disarm implants by calling in frequencies that are the complete opposite. When we deliver these opposite frequencies directly into the implants, their tiny circuits burn out and they are no longer viable. Removal isn't really necessary as long as they are disengaged.

The most important thing to remember about abductees is that if they know they are being abducted, the feeling is often like the rape victim who fears the rapist may come back and harm her at any time. The difference is that once the rapist is jailed, the victim can relax and know that she is safe. An abductee is dealing with a situation that is insurmountable in a sense of reality. Since the perpetrators are otherworldly and so far impossible to catch, the abductee lives in fear of abduction over and over again, knowing that it can happen at any time and there is no control over it.

CHAPTER TEN

The Healing Session

When we return back into universal harmonization, there is a momentary bump in our energy system as it reboots. Then, we begin to pulse with the rhythm of timelessness and our healthfulness returns. The multi-dimensional healing session is a sacred rite. It is at once complex and simple. It is a privilege and an honor to merge with the field of another human being, for they and their life force, the myriad layers that compose them, are expressions of creation manifested as a reflection of itself. In a way, each of us is an aspect of God. Each time I have encountered the complex intricate workings of another, I have stood in awe at their beauty, perfection, and the dysfunction that can occur.

Having accessed literally thousands of multi-dimensional fields over the years, I have learned on one hand that there are predictable patterns, and on another hand, that no two beings are put together the same. Every session brings new awareness and sometimes surprises that are beyond imagining. As I have worked, I have realized that certain movements or tiny gestures could completely change the experience and its outcome.

In this chapter I have broken down the many aspects of the healing session so that you, the reader, can learn to experience the myriad intricacies that are the healing. Learning what is in this chapter won't give you enough information or experience to hang out a shingle. It takes tons of practice to realize the gentle power that the healer who wields these skills has when merged with the field system of another human being. But this is a good start. When we realize that we hold the power of creation in our very being, we can begin to become aware of how touching the light within others can literally change tissues, energy fields, and even the lives our clients are living.

I have broken this part of the book into sections of importance and finally illustrated a basic healing session. Each section will give you valuable knowledge toward understanding the intricacies of yourself and your clients.

Mudras and Their Effect on Our Body Frequencies

When I first started working with energy, strange movements began to happen spontaneously with my hands and fingers. When I was alone, both hands moved into unusual positions of their own accord. Later, when I began touching the bodies of others, as one hand encountered the body, my other hand formed these strange positions. If I moved my hand just a little bit in one direction or another, up, down, forward, back, I could feel the energy change inside of me. Sometimes as my hands moved even subtly, they and my fingers changed into different positions.

I noticed that when I touched certain parts of my client's bodies, my remaining hand nearly always formed into these odd positions. Later still, I realized that my hands were automatically changing into Mudras.

In Sanskrit, *mudra* means "seal." Mudras are positions of the hands and, sometimes even the body, which have an effect on the energy in and around us as well as how we feel emotionally. As we form mudras, the flow of energy in the inner pathways of our bodies is opened, enhanced, or allowed to build up, making corrections to our various body systems. Using the mudras locks in these subtle changes until we stop doing them. A brain study was published in the National Academy of Sciences in November 2009, which discovered that mudras stimulate the same regions in the brain as language.

Mudras have been used for untold years in Buddhist and Hindu practices as well as in martial arts, yoga, and in other sectors of belief and practice. When applied to the self, major changes can occur in health, awareness, intellect, intuition, and virtually every part of our human experience. When we are joined with the energy field of another and we apply mudras, they can reap similar benefits. Remember, when we join energy fields with another, we both experience many of the same things.

I never knew what these amazing positions were called, or that they even had names. Like the meridian points, I had complete faith that what I was doing was important and there was no question it was effective!

Many of my students have found their hands acting of their own accord as well and have been able to successfully utilize the mudras without needing to know what they were about. In the interest of giving fuller information here, I wanted to include at least some of these powerful yet subtle hand and finger movements to give the reader an idea of what is happening. If you want to have more understanding about mudras, many great books and videos are available that can teach you more specifically. I find that when I get too left-brained, needing to know or understand, my process becomes less effective and the healing work becomes diluted by my brain activity.

In any case, I present here some of the more common ones with their appropriate names and applications. There are many more. If you practice with these, use both hands always. As you do, try moving your hands very slowly farther away or closer to you, to the right or left, and see how you feel inside when you do. If you are paying attention, you will be amazed at how the tiniest movement can change the entire feeling of the energy within you! If you find your hands moving of their own accord, you may discover other mudras on your own!

Surya Mudra

Directions: Bend the ring finger down and press it gently to the hand with the thumb.

Effects of this mudra include:

- Enhancing thyroid energy

- Reducing cholesterol levels in the body

- Helping to reduce weight

- Reducing anxiety

- Assisting in correction of indigestion problems

Prana Mudra

Directions: Bend the ring and little fingers down and touch their tips with the tip of the thumb, keeping the remaining two fingers stretched up straight. *Improves overall body strength and vitality.*

Effects of this mudra include:

- Strengthening the immune system

- Improving eye acuity and reducing eye-related diseases

- Assisting with vitamin deficiency and fatigue

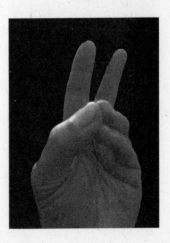

Apan Vayu Mudra

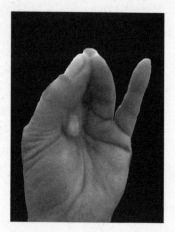

Description: Fold the forefinger to touch the soft mound below the thumb. The little finger should be held straight up. Then place tips of middle and ring finger together on the very tip of the thumb so they are all touching each other.

Effects of this Mudra include:

- Strengthening the heart

- Can be used as emergency first aid for severe heart attack (only if administered within the first two seconds)

- Boosting self-confidence

- Can assist in normalizing blood pressure

- Can stop vomiting

- Assisting with problems related to menstruation

- Purifying the entire body

Gyan Mudra

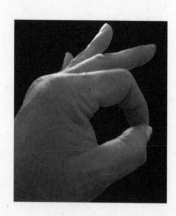

Description: The thumb and index finger come together gently touching tip to tip while all of the other fingers remain upright.

Effects of this Mudra include:

- Establishing a sense of mental peace

- Increasing concentration

- Sharpening the memory

- Bringing a sense of spirituality

- Helping to cure insomnia

- Soothing mental disorders

- Alleviating stress

- Alleviating depression

- Overcoming drowsiness

- Developing telepathic abilities

- Developing clairvoyant and extra-sensory abilities

Rudra Mudra

Description: Bring tips of index and ring fingers together onto the tip of the thumb, with other fingers extended straight up.

Effects of this mudra include:

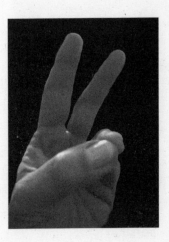

- Alleviating dizziness

- Improving blood circulation

- Bringing clarity to thought

- Lowering blood pressure

- Improving eyesight

- Improving breathing

- Helping to control eating habits

- Assisting with blocked veins

- Improving concentration

Apana Mudra

Description: Touch the tips of the thumb, middle and ring fingers.

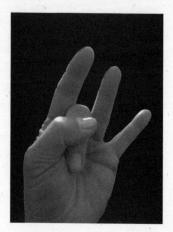

Effects of this mudra include:

- Adjustments to liver

- Adjustments to gall bladder

- Assisting in removal of waste products

- Affecting toxic release

- Assisting with bladder problems

- Helping to balance the mind

- Improving self confidence

- Helping instill patience

- Establishing serenity and achieving inner harmony

Prithvi Mudra

Description: Place the tip of the ring finger onto the mound below the thumb. Extend all the other fingers straight up and keep them comfortably as straight as possible.

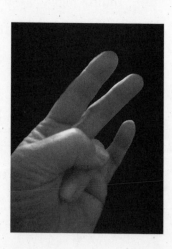

Effects of this mudra include:

- Assisting liver health

- Creating inner stability

- Achieving self-assurance

- Assisting stomach health

- Strengthening body and mind

- Bringing a glow to the skin

- Increasing energy

Varuna Mudra

Description: Lay the thumb down over the top of the little finger at the second joint. Keep the remaining three fingers comfortably straight.

Effects of this mudra include:

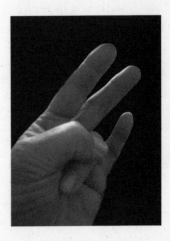

- Enhancing beauty

- Removal of impurities from the blood

- Helping restore moisture to the skin

- Relieving painful cramps

Shunya Mudra

Description: Place thumb down over top of the ring finger between the first and second joints. Keep the remaining three fingers straight.

Effects of this mudra include:

- Helping heal earaches

- Treating deafness

- Helping alleviate vertigo

- Curing numbness in the body

Vayu Mudra

Description: Place thumb across the top of the index finger just below the first joint. Keep the other three fingers straight.

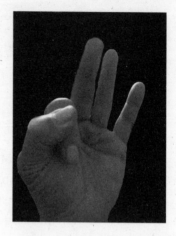

Effects of this mudra include:

- Alleviating rheumatism

- Helping relieve sciatica

- Helping loosen a stiff neck

- Reducing knee pain

- Relieving gout

- Reducing joint pain in the hands and feet

- Helping cure paralysis

- Calming hysteria

Surabhi Mudra

Description: Join the little and ring fingers, then join the middle and index fingers together and spread them apart in a V formation.

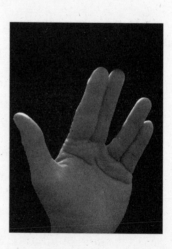

Effects of this mudra include:

- Reducing rheumatic inflammation

- Sharpening your brain power

Hands On: A Step By Step Methodology to Access, Read, Interpret, and Correct the Anomalies within an Etheric Field

Entering into the healing space is like walking into the most sacred temple in creation. It is also a process. The following sections will take you step-by-step into the Holy of Holies, the healing mergence of you and your subject.

Setting the Space

Setting a proper environment is a must. When the client first walks into our space, whether it is our home, an office, or a room, that space should be uncluttered, welcoming, clean, and calm. Our cell phones, beepers, and other electronic apparatus should be turned off.

Speaking of electronics, it is highly recommended that we keep our computers, cell phones, and other electronic devices in another room away from where we are practicing. Why? Simply because the kinds of energy we will be working with are strong enough to fry computer chips and other fragile electronic parts. Over the years, I have seen this many times. The worst was when I was working to improve the hearing of a friend who was going deaf. As I worked energetically inside her ears, both of her hearing aids were fried. Fortunately, they were under warranty. When she took them in to the technician to be fixed, they were irreparable. The tech wanted to know what she had been doing, as he had never seen anything like it!

This warning also goes for pacemakers and other implanted items that may be in the body. Always ask if there are any of those kinds of items in the body and if so, in cases such as hearing aids, ask the client to remove them. In the case of implanted electronics, we *must inform the client* that energy work can affect them.

If the client still wants to have the session, then it is best to avoid the particular area of the implanted device. We can still have the same results by directing intention instead of a stream of intense energy to that specific area.

Etheric healing should be done in a private, quiet place. Music is great in the background, but not if we are singing along with it. Best to use something that is for relaxation or mood setting. I absolutely do *not* recommend hemi-sync music during these sessions because this kind of recording contains frequencies that initiate specific types of brain waves. Usually, the frequencies of energy and brain wave patterns we use when we work multi-dimensionally are far above those that are used in hemi-sync, so playing hemi-sync during a healing session can limit or vary the results.

Also keep in mind that many people are allergic to fragrances and perfumes, so colognes, oils, scented candles, or anything that has a fragrance should be eliminated from the room. Aromatherapy oils and other similar products also carry harmonic frequencies that may be disharmonic to the Etheric work you are creating and so should not be used in this modality.

A quiet place to work is an absolute must. There should be nothing going on in the background or immediately outside the room to distract either the healer or the client.

Once the session begins and we merge with the Etheric field of our clients, we should not interrupt the session for anything short of a disaster. Interruptions affect the client's experience, our levels of concentration as healers, and even the movement of energies.

Privacy is paramount to a professional environment. Make sure that whoever might be in the waiting area cannot hear the conversational exchanges between you and your current client. If necessary, place a fan, music, or a sound machine in the waiting room to help defray sounds from the healing room.

The Power of Emotion: Our Own and Our Client's

Once we have accessed the Etheric field of another being, a multitude of experiences awaits us. We may find anomalies in different levels of the field, in or on the Etheric bodies, densities, inflammations of energies, and even outright junk that has been picked up on various levels of reality. We may also have emotional responses to what we encounter. We must remember that our emotional responses are *reactive*. They are *not* usually our emotions, but an *empathic response* to the client's experiences. Emotions are imprinted in the Etheric field and can really pack a wallop.

For example, I worked with a young woman who lived over three thousand miles away. Her mom referred her to me. I talked with the girl the week before our scheduled healing session to make sure that she really wanted me to work with her and to establish what issues she wanted assistance with. I had a great feel for her after our conversation and felt that the session was going to be a pretty tame adventure.

The following week, I tuned into her long distance, and as soon as I accessed her Etheric field, I was nearly thrown backward by the extent of trauma that I felt in her system. It was massive, fresh, and powerful. As I worked on her, I concentrated on relieving her system of the trauma. Powerful emotions swept through me as I worked. I cried. I felt shame, anger, and many other feelings nearly all at once. The emotions and the damage to her field were so fresh and intense I could barely stay with it.

After I finished the session, I called the young woman.

"What happened to you since we talked? Something terrible! There was so much trauma it was hard to work. . . ."

"Yes," she said, "Right after we talked last week I was raped in my back yard. He was waiting for me when I went out the back door. It was awful. . . ."

I really hated hearing that. Unfortunately, now everything that I had felt during our session made sense. What she was carrying around with her was a nightmare. He had hit her out of nowhere, and she was terrified that he would come back again.

I was able to ascertain that she had been so ashamed of what happened that she hadn't told anyone about the attack. Fortunately, after talking her through some of her feelings, I was able to convince her to hang up with me and to call her mom immediately. She did and was then able to get some real help with what had happened.

Trauma in another person's field feels to me like being plugged straight into an electrical socket. My insides light up and the energy feels immense, as if it is building and could explode at any minute. It is much like an internal electrical shock and feels like physical anxiousness.

The more recently the trauma has occurred, the greater its intensity. Sometimes we feel trauma in our hands when we first touch the body. Trauma feels chaotic, intense, and foreign to the overall energy field. In a way, trauma is like feelings that have no logical place in the mind, so instead they run rampant through the body and energy field looking for where they fit. The problem is that those feelings don't fit in our everyday reality so they remain as static in our energy fields.

Other emotions can hit us just as hard. Grief is a great one to cause spontaneous tears. Guilt is another, and of course there are many different emotions that are just as powerful and can show up when we least expect them. Conversely, we might feel positive emotions too, but it is usually the negative ones that have been stuffed down into the consciousness and the body that can sneak up on us like cosmic two by fours.

Trauma may also be of a physical nature, and so we might feel it anywhere in or on the body. If there is an area of injury, for instance, a broken leg that healed long ago, the limb may still carry the trauma of the actual event. We can alleviate trauma by draining it out of the field or by transmuting that energy into normal energy for whatever area we have accessed.

Sometimes when we are working with another person, we may feel these traumas as if they are our own. This phenomenon alone is one of the reasons we must be very familiar with our own issues and have worked through them before we ever work on anyone else. It is also why we should never commiserate with our clients. Comparing notes and experiences when another person is in that kind of distress only serves to make things worse. Instead of feeling validated, they feel like they haven't been heard. Our clients didn't come to hear our problems; they came for help with theirs.

Over the years I found that having dealt with my own issues and perhaps having had similar experiences to those of some of my clients, I have been able to forthrightly give good, calm, and responsible assistance to them rather than getting caught up in the drama of their experiences. I am also able to bring forth great depths of compassion because I honestly do know how my clients feel. Being able to look someone in the eye and say, "Yes, I do understand," and mean it is a priceless asset in the healer's toolbox.

Compassion is one of the greatest gifts a healer can give to her client. Compassion is a form of love, and when we fuel the energy that is coming through us to our clients with love and compassion, the results are always more profound.

After we have worked with a client, it is a great idea to take time for ourselves to make sure we have retained our balance and not "taken on" any of our client's stuff. Some of the experiences we have while we are enmeshed with our client's energy fields can be difficult to distinguish in terms of who is feeling what. Practice definitely helps with this, but, as I said, having a good handle on our own stuff goes a long way in maintaining that balance.

Before the Session: Consider How Our Clients May React to Etheric Healing

Touching the light is an intangible form of healing. To many who are encountering it for the first time, it is a "woo woo" scary experience because this kind of healing is far from the considered norm. It is always a great idea to take time with new clients to fully explain the process and benefits (not every detail, just an informal outline). Tell them that the work, because it is multi-dimensional in nature, can have both immediate and long-term effects.

When we work in the Etheric fields, sometimes it takes a little while for the changes to reach our current reality. Because of that, I tell my clients that this kind of healing has trickle down effects that may go on for days, weeks, or even months. It is also a good idea to explain to the client that having any other kind of energy work for at least a month after your session together is not a good idea, as the effects are continually in occurrence.

Never be in a rush to get someone on the table. The client really needs to have a trusting relationship with the healer so that they can both believe and accept the healing that they have requested.

Some healers have animals, such as a dog or cat, present in the healing room because they feel the animal contributes to the healing. Personally, I find this a distraction. Animals love the energy work and will bask in it. They also add yet another set of biological frequencies in the room that can confuse the situation in subtle ways. Sometimes critters want to become involved and will jump onto the client during very sensitive times. Other animals may be so sensitive to the work that they will act differently or do things they might not otherwise do during a session. Also, some clients may have allergy issues around animals.

Finally, we must be balanced in every way and leave our personal issues at the door before entering into a session with anyone. If something is happening in our life that day that affects our ability to be fully present with the client, our energy levels, or our emotional state on a particular day, it is best to reschedule the session to another day or time.

During the Session

During the session, the client may experience any number of sensations, visions, emotions, or other strange phenomena that he is not used to or hasn't had before. This is very normal.

A client may become very cold or, conversely, extremely warm as the energy frequencies change during the session. It is a great idea to have a blanket nearby or to offer it before we begin the actual session. Energy fluctuations can be quite subtle or profound, depending upon what is being corrected or changed in the system.

Everyone reacts to subtle energy work differently. Some people just zone out, becoming extremely relaxed or even out of body temporarily, and they are very comfortable with that. Others have involuntary reactions in their bodies. Their hands may move involuntarily, their bodies may twitch with energy changes or even writhe in response to the energies. Some people actually thrash around with the energies. If that is the case, in my opinion, there is some resistance on some level, and I will stop and ask the client to breathe and relax with the energies, to let herself be carried by the energies. This will usually calm the reactions.

As different areas of energy open up, are reconnected, or are changed, energy begins to rush through areas that had previously been stalled. As this occurs, the energy may reach yet another blockage and, not often, but possibly, cause pain. This pain is nothing more than blocked energy. If this occurs, just ask the body where to touch so that the blockage can be alleviated, and let your hands and fingers connect the places. Once you do, the pain almost instantly subsides.

Another possibility for the client is that she may begin to see colors, shapes, or even have visions during sessions. She may even become aware of what you are doing in her Etheric field. This new opening can be very exciting for the client to say the least. It is important to educate the client about what is happening so that she can gain a sense of normalcy for her experiences rather than to be afraid of them.

Emotional releases are almost a given during these kinds of sessions. Many people cry involuntarily and don't even know why. When this happens, it is nothing more than hidden emotion releasing from the body. The emotion is released with the energy changes and rises to the surface like a bubble. As it reaches the surface and the so-called bubble of energy pops, emotions are experienced. At other times the client will feel blissful or a profound sense of oneness with creation.

Negative emotions can arise as well, and when they do, I generally encourage my clients to say what they didn't, feel what they hadn't allowed, or whatever applies to that moment.

Some clients are very verbal during releases, shouting or even screaming from the intensity of their withheld emotions. Vocal expression can run the gamut in the healing room. There is nothing in particular that we need to do about that except to be strongly supportive. If the client is holding back, re-stuffing the emotions as they attempt to rise out of the body, I usually stop and ask him to let things flow so that he is finally finished with the pain. Once the client has permission, he usually will let go.

It can be very easy for the healer, in an effort to console the client, to want to spontaneously throw your body over him in a huge hug. This isn't advised and could be misinterpreted by the client in a number of ways. We tend to want to be empathetic when people become emotional, but in the healing session, expressions of pain are the perfect release, and we must simply and unconditionally be witnesses for this. A simple touch of the hand validates the client and shows her that we are there.

Communicating to the client what is happening during a session can be accomplished in a couple of ways. We can talk to the client as we work, which, honestly, I find distracting because when we are immersed in the Etheric field, there is a lot going on that requires our attention. Alternatively, we can simply keep track of what we have changed, the impressions we have received during the session, and whatever has occurred, and tell these things to the client after the session is over and he is fully back in his body.

After the Session

Communication about the session is vital. The client has come for assistance and should be given a responsible non-dramatic honest assessment of the session. What was found, what was done, and how he can participate to maintain the healing that was done.

Sometimes we pick up ongoing patterns and issues that are affecting everything the client does so it is best to make the client responsible for changing those patterns by educating her about them. Usually the client will laugh and agree that the issue is both real and a problem. Once they are more aware of the extent of the effect that the pattern is having, clients often seriously participate on their own behalf. I usually tell them this is their homework and that if they don't do it, the work that we have just done will ultimately return to dysfunction in their systems. It is true!

Touching the light can have a powerful effect on our clients and us as well. The client may feel spaced out, disoriented, or in a state of bliss after the session. I always laughingly tell my clients that the effects of this kind of treatment are better than drugs. It is true!

The reason that our clients are so affected is that we have literally changed their entire system balance, and that can be temporarily disorienting. If your client is one who becomes very disoriented, make quite sure that you give him plenty of water and have him sit until he is safe to stand; then have him sit in the waiting room or a quiet place until it is safe for him to drive.

Driving immediately after this kind of session can be the same as driving while under the influence of drugs or alcohol. Men tend to get far more spaced out than women for some reason. Even if the client insists he is fine, get him to sit anyway for at least a little while until you are sure he is okay to drive. This effect usually only lasts less than an hour until the client gets used to the new state of balance.

Before clients leave, tell them what they can expect. Etheric healing can affect everyone differently. If there was a lot of work done around emotional issues and energies were rearranged, any time from immediately after the session to within three days later, the client may have a huge release, or what I call crash and burn, for a few days. This is actually normal and is a very good thing. The release can be intense and powerful, with huge emotions of various kinds surfacing. Tell clients that if this occurs to let the emotions out. Once they do, they are finished with them and won't have ongoing problems from them because the emotions will have dissipated out of the body and the Etheric field.

After the session, clients usually will sleep exceedingly well that night, or within a few days, they will need to isolate, just be still and away from everyone for a day or so. This too is a common reaction.

People are quite used to doctors and other practitioners telling them that they need repeat sessions. When we perform Etheric work, if it is thorough, they may never need us again. Or, like the layers of an onion, other issues may show up later. What I tell my clients is that whether or not they need to return is completely *their* decision (unless the situation is an acute injury that could benefit from repeated treatments). If they continue to improve and then plateau without reaching their full desired effects, I suggest they may choose to return. Or, if they experience good results and then begin to backslide, I suggest they may want to revisit. In any case except an acute injury, working with someone less than a month after our previous session is kind of redundant because the energies we left at work during our previous session are still in progress. Sometimes the energies are still changing long after we have done the actual work so we can't see or sense accurately what needs to be done next.

Anomalies in the Etheric Anatomy

There seems to be no limit to what we may encounter in the energy fields of others. There are some pretty common anomalies though that we will most definitely encounter on a regular basis. Anomalies take on countless forms and can either be easily removed or can be extremely resistant.

Some resist because they are parasitic and derive their life force from our energy fields while others are resistant because they have been instilled by the hidden emotions or traumatic experiences and even beliefs of our clients. Here are some of the more common ones:

The Etheric Burr

The burr-shaped anomaly is most often found attached to the external field. It is a parasitic attachment that either can cause energy to leak out of the exterior field or can cause thickening of the field wall like a scar on skin. This kind of anomaly may cause chronic illness or pain or low physical energy, and once it is removed and destroyed, the illness or pain generally ceases altogether and energy levels rise.

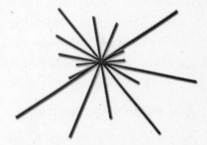

Burr-like anomaly is often found in the exterior field.

Cylindrical Blockages and Implants

Cylindrical anomalies are generally on the interior of a field and can be found anywhere in the system. They can be any size and are usually a form of blockage but can occasionally be found as implants too. When the cylinders are a blockage, they are heavy feeling and dark gray or brown, sometimes even black. When in the form of an implant they are entirely energetic, comprising frequencies that are different from the client's system but so closely harmonized that they are easy to miss. When they are implants in energy form, they are usually bright green, and they feel much lighter in weight. These can be extracted from their area of embedment and destroyed.

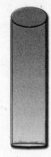

Cylindrical
blockage.

Disk-Shaped Blockages and Implants

The disk shaped blockage is another parasitic form of energy that becomes embedded in most any level of the Etheric field. If found in the physical body, disks are usually in the chest or torso and rarely, but on occasion, on the bottoms of the feet.

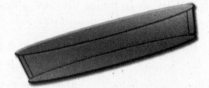

Disk-like blockage.

Disks can also be an energetic implant, which may act in a number of ways such as gathering information about the system of its victim, sending information into the field to effect change in the frequencies or energy interactions, or even to act as transmitters of information to and from the victim from an unknown source.

When the disk is a blockage, it is most often dark gray or brown but can occasionally be black, and when it is an implant, it is usually a group of particles that have come together to form the disk. These are bright green.

Rod-Shaped Anomalies

Rod type anomalies can be found most anywhere in the system and come in virtually any color. They also often come in multiples that may be of different colors. When they are positioned in relation to the physical body, the rod is generally impaled through the body, and the victim often suffers chronic pain and occasionally disease in that area. When the rod or rods are removed, usually the symptoms disappear.

Rods also come in a tiny form of crystallized energy that is thorn-like and can act as an irritant to the field where it is found. In this smaller form, rods are most often found inside the solar plexus vortex. This is because the solar plexus is where energies from others and our environment enter our system. When those energies are disharmonic, they become crystallized and become lodged in the walls of our various energy levels or forms and act as irritants that cause pain, inflammation, organ dysfunction, or other issues.

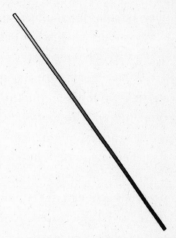

Rod shaped crystallized energy can be any size or location in the Etheric anatomy and often causes chronic pain.

Blockages

Blockages are the most prevalent anomaly found in any energy system on any level. They can be of any shape or size and range from nearly transparent to practically manifested dense matter. Blockages cause the energy field to malfunction in many different ways. They can completely stop the flow of energy or

Blockages can be any size, density or shape, and can occur at any level around, on, or within the Etheric anatomy.

cause it to reroute to completely avoid the blocked area. When this happens, the blocked area becomes painful or dysfunctional, even diseased. Blockages can be removed from the body and destroyed or can usually be alleviated with either the command to DECOMPRESS or to DISSIPATE.

Thought Forms

Thought forms are always found in the external field and can range from inanimate to mimicking living objects or forms. These forms are most often symbolic to the client and represent some perceived reality. Thought forms represent fervent beliefs that affect our behaviors and our perceptions to our very cores. In a way, thought forms are energetic doppelgangers of our fears. They often take on a fiendish behavior that is usually more mischievous than anything.

Thought forms are disruptive to the overall energy system because they can move around like living things in the external field, changing the energy relationships and flow patterns.

Basically, thought forms are fears that have become so real that they take on not only a persona, but also a manifested reality that becomes active in the system. These can be easily removed and transmuted into either inert matter or source energy.

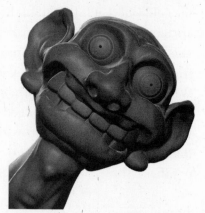

There are, of course, many other types of anomalies from countless sources, different affectations that have unpredictable behaviors which can be found in the various Etheric systems of humanity. The important thing to remember is to stay out of our imaginations, deal with these things as they present, have a sense of humor, and deal with them strongly and surely in each case. The truth is that we don't have to imagine anything. The reality of what happens outside of our local reality is strange enough!

Thought forms can look quite scary and act very real. Thought forms can take any form or reality, depending upon the fear that drives them. They are always found in the exterior field and can be still or quite animated and are the product of our fears.

Making Changes in the Etheric Fields

I have found when teaching this modality that one word commands alleviate the possibilities for error and will bring about exactly what we mean. Just like when we create reality with pure intention, when we use too many commands, too many words or thoughts or even intentions, instead of correcting problems, we can scramble the energies or, worse, bring on an effect that we did not intend. To best learn to effect change in an energy system, specific commands are paramount to the healer's skill set.

When we make a command using a specific word to make a change, the energies will follow the command and do exactly what is needed without further instructions. Reality really does follow intention.

The statement above is the most important thing to remember when doing this kind of healing work. The energy already knows what to do; basically all we need to do is direct it.

The next most important thing to remember is:

Never, ever, force change!

Forcing change can have drastically undesirable results! For instance, in one of my classes I had paired my students up so that they could begin having practical experience with the work. I had taught them how to make commands in a clear and concise manner.

One of the students misread what she was sensing in her partner's energy field. She was at a crucial part of the session, having raised the Etheric bodies up to work on them. Her partner had left her body, which is common during this phase of the treatment. The student who was in the healer's position made a command to correct what she thought needed to happen and there was no change. Instead of questioning her perception, she thought there was resistance so she commanded the change again only this time with a powerful force. Unfortunately, what she had sensed was completely inaccurate and because she had commanded a powerful force of energy to work on a misperception, strange things occurred immediately!

Unbeknownst to her, her partner had had a serious traumatic childhood event during which her energy field had fragmented. The fragmented aspect was vulnerable because the Etheric bodies were exposed and she was out of her body. In other words her consciousness was free floating at the moment the command was made. Instead of the intended repair happening, the partner's consciousness was jolted into the wrong aspect of herself, and so instead of making a minor repair, my student inadvertently jerked her partner's consciousness into the aspect of the seven-year-old child! And there it stayed.

I saw it happen but wasn't sure what I was seeing at first. The subject sat straight up and had the most innocent, childish expression on her face. She asked to go to the restroom and when she came back she went and curled up in a chair like a scared child. She spoke like a child, her posturing was that of a child, and she was terrified, not understanding what had happened to her!

After fully assessing the situation I realized what had happened and was able to fix the problem, but it was a pretty scary few moments for them both. I realized in that moment that as a teacher I really needed to make clearer that the power of these commands is infinite and immediate and so they should be used with ease and grace and never, ever, forced. I also learned a lot about consciousness and its intricacies that day. That event opened a whole new can of worms that I could relate to mental health issues such as multiple personality disorders, post traumatic stress syndrome, and even schizophrenia as well as other less disabling problems.

Sometimes we will notice resistance in an area of an energy field. There may be instances when the energy seems to begin to change and then goes back to its dysfunction, or it refuses to change at all. In these cases, either there is resistance on the part of the client to let go of those particular injuries or issues, or there is something else somewhere in the energy field that we need to find and correct before we can make that particular change.

Just because one area is dysfunctional does not mean that that dysfunction is the root cause of the problem. Remember that the body tells a story, as does the energy system as a whole, so if we find an anomaly in one area, chances are that there will be other affectations in related areas. There is always a pattern of dysfunction, and once it is repaired on all levels, the problem may disappear completely or at least greatly improve.

How to Command Changes

When we are merged with the field of another, the slightest intention or thought can bring about change. We must be careful to cause only the necessary alteration and nothing more. Making changes in the Etheric field can be done easily with one-word commands. Each word is a powerful and unmistakable instruction that will alter the state of the intended area and even the entire field structure. Adding other words muddies the command and leaves greater room for unintentional change that can be detrimental to the subject. In this mergence, a highly sensitive environment, errors can be unforgivable!

Using the Basic Commands

When we work within the Etheric field of another, we don't ask for change, we command it. We do so with our hearts and only positive intentions. Those intentions do not need to be specific, just pure.

Following are the basic commands that you can use when merged with the field of another. Remember that these should never be forced. If you meet resistance in any area with any command, try it gently another time or two and if the desired change still doesn't occur, leave that area for the time being and keep working. Sometimes change occurs much easier when we go back to an area later, or the repair may occur spontaneously after something else in another area of the field is corrected. Remember that everything interrelates no matter how it may seem. Everything that you do anywhere in someone's Etheric anatomy affects the entirety of their being.

As you become more proficient as a healer using this method, you may come up with commands that fit situations that I haven't mentioned here. That is fine, just remember, no matter what, to keep them simple, limit them to one word if you can, don't invest a lot of thought trying to analyze your perceptions of your clients, and trust your guidance as well as your intuition!

When using the following commands, it is vitally important to use the single words and let the energy system interpret how to use them on its own. We don't need to have specific intentions with these commands, because the Etheric anatomy will respond perfectly as the commands are given. If we add extra meanings to these commands in any way, the outcome of their use is changed drastically, so it is best to let them speak for themselves and let the energy in its respective areas of the Etheric anatomy respond because it knows exactly what to do once reminded.

Here are the basic commands:

- **ALIGN or STRAIGHTEN** (whichever best applies): There are multiple lines of energy running through the body, such as the pranic tube and the meridian lines. Sometimes these get skewed, becoming diagonally aligned because a blockage has pushed them out of alignment or some other anomaly has caused them to reroute. If you just use the STRAIGHTEN command, the line of energy will straighten where it is and not necessarily where it belongs. The most preferred command is ALIGN, because then not only will the energy line straighten, it will move back into its correct position. If the energy line does not reposition and then stay with the change, there is likely some reason, such as a blockage or an inflamed area that is pushing the line out of place and so must be taken care of first.

- **CENTER:** Sometimes an area, a line of energy, a chakra, or an Etheric body will be off center. This command requires that the aspect of the Etheric anatomy return to its exact center position.

- **DECOMPRESS:** When we encounter blockages or densities of energy, this command causes the blockage or density to loosen up and return to normal levels of density.

- **DISSIPATE:** After decompression, there may be dense particles left in the area. Using this command causes the field to release the dense particles where they will return to perfect light energy. This command also works well to relieve inflamed energy in overcharged areas.

- **CLARIFY:** On every level of the Etheric anatomy, there can be different issues regarding the harmonics. Each area has its own particular set of harmonics that is unique to that area but may for different reasons become confused in patterning or become of different, mixed sets of harmonics that cause problems virtually anywhere. When we use this command, the field is required to unify to its normal state.

- **EQUALIZE:** This is another but more powerful version of CLARIFY. When the movement of energy has gotten erratic in patterning or direction or there are densities, for example, in one of the Etheric bodies, this command is a sure and fast way to make all of the necessary corrections with one command.

- **ROOT:** This command applies to chakras only. Often a chakra will become angulated, pulling away from its connection to the body. At other times a chakra will become misplaced, rising above the body or sinking downward into the body. Once you have repositioned the chakra, command that it root, and it will reattach at exact center and plane where it should be.

- **CALIBRATE:** This command has multiple uses. It can change size, density, oscillation (which is the rate of spin of the vortexes), and many other more subtle issues. For instance, if a chakra is too long or too short, if an Etheric body, particularly the emotional body, is too large or small, if the external field has mixed frequencies and there is chaos in the field, when we calibrate any of these errors, the field is instantly normalized, the size is corrected, and correct movement is established. Also if the chakra isn't spinning correctly or at all, calibrating it will instigate the oscillation of spin and then correct the speed of the spin.

- **REPAIR:** Sometimes there are tears in the walls of a field that cause energy leakages or damage to the area. This command takes care of any degree of tearing or damage to any field or body on any level.

- **TRANSMUTE:** This is a vitally important command with many purposes and one of the most powerful that we can use because using it is literally commanding that something change form completely.

  When we find something that does not belong in someone's Etheric field system or if we find areas of energy that are dysfunctional, damaged, stagnant, or have other problems, this command tells the energy of that area to return to its normal set of frequencies. The light within the energy remembers its original form and so when commanded will return to that state.

  This command can also be used on items that are removed from the field to destroy them. When transmuting items one of two things generally happens: Either the item changes into pure light energy where it will be used by creation for some other purpose or it will turn into inert matter, which is basically cosmic dust.

- **REMOVE:** When we find foreign affectations, energy formations that do not belong in the field of our subject, they need to be removed from the Etheric anatomy. This command causes the object to become released from the field. It is often used in conjunction with DISSIPATE or TRANSMUTE because, once removed, the object must be destroyed so that it does not reattach.

- **ASSIMILATE:** When fragmentation of chakras, energies, or our inter-dimensional aspects has occurred, this command calls in all parts of the fragments and requires that they reconstruct into the proper form or harmonization. This command is most often, but not limited to, being used for bringing harmonic alignment of the Etheric aspects and for putting the throat or solar plexus vortexes back together after they have fragmented.

- **ATTUNE:** Once we have finished making all required repairs in an area we must use this command so that the area becomes harmonized in its proper frequency sets in connection with the rest of the Etheric anatomy. We should always use this command as the last one in any area.

Basic Order of Touch for the Seventh Sense Healing Process

Now that we have a good basic understanding and awareness of how to merge and work within an Etheric field and what we might encounter there, we are ready to learn how to perform a basic Seventh Sense Attunement. Below are complete step by step and illustrated instructions about how to easily work within the Etheric anatomy.

Remember always that there is a human being in your hands, and that when doing this, you are merged on every level of reality with your subject. Be compassionate. Be love. Be unconditional and lack judgment. Tell the truth without drama and trauma and give your client possibilities, not your idea of what their life should look like. Remember that every human being has the ability and the possibility to make a different choice in his life.

I decided to share this basic session instruction because this stuff really works. I am sharing it, however, with a few caveats. First of all, the work may seem simple and easy, but it is the most powerful modality I have ever encountered. Please, please, be careful of what you command and keep your imagination at bay. An active imagination can cause more damage than good when working in the Etheric realms. They are strange enough without us adding to them!

Also, sharing this information here does not give the reader permission to hang a shingle or to teach this modality without complete instruction and written permission from the author. Believe it or not, this information is only basic to what might be found or encountered by an unprepared practitioner, and my interest is about the safety of you and your clients.

Always and only have permission from your client personally. Don't just ask their "higher self" because nine point nine times out of ten the answer you hear will be rooted in your own desire to help someone. We must always have *direct* permission to work with anyone no matter what. I do make exceptions for people's young children or for a spouse whose other half cannot speak for himself but rarely others. This work is a complete mergence within the being of another soul, and entering there without permission is not okay. It is far worse than walking into a stranger's house uninvited.

These pages are meant as a guideline for remembering the order of repairs in a healing session and are no way meant to be or imply a session in its entirety. In reality, each session is different and one may feel a need to vary from this outline. That is fine as long as there is a conscious effort to maintain balance for the client in that process!

There are several levels to this technique. Please do not vary from the order in which they are given. Each precedes the other for a reason and builds on the one before it. If you find that new or different one word commands would be more adequate or appropriate than the ones I have given, use them. If you are drawn to touch an area different than I have shown, touch it. Just keep the sequence in order and remember when you are done to separate out of your client's energy field.

Mostly, follow your heart, never your head, and let the energy go where it will. It knows what to do. It is part of our source and has the memory of all time within it.

With all that being said, here are full instructions:

Level One

(Remember throughout the session, when you follow this touch pattern, to remain with your hands in place until you feel, sense, or see a shift under or in your hands. Also, remember to counter your touch by touching at least one other area of the body!) Use your guidance and don't resist moving your touch to another area if so guided.

General Balancing

The first level is a basic and general balancing that gives overall quick balance to the energy system. This balancing is not specific but is vital to how the different levels of the system respond during the rest of the session. This balancing also, in a way, alerts the multi-dimensional levels of the system to become accessible to the healer. The step one balancing literally opens a portal to access the different layers and levels of the Etheric anatomy:

1. Approach the client; ask permission to touch him.

2. Place your hands above and parallel with the face. (What do you feel? What is your sense?) Allow the energy to build up between your hands until you have a ball of energy there.

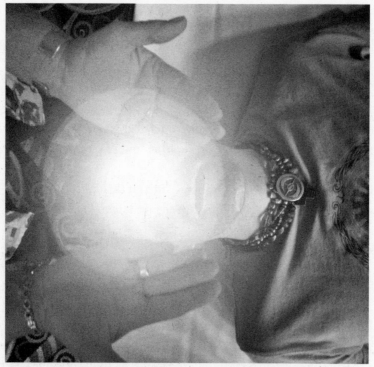

As the energy builds in our hands, an orb of light forms, carrying our consciousness with it. Let the energy between your hands expand.

3. Once you feel that the ball of energy is stable between your hands, lower your hands to either side of your client's head. This is when mergence occurs and you begin to access his energy field. Be patient until you feel the balance. Once you have, then begin the session.

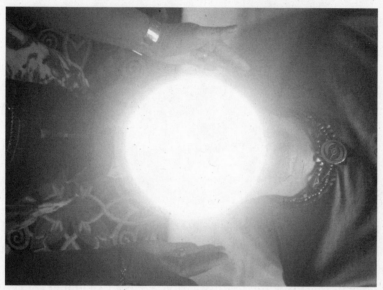

When mergence occurs the orb of light becomes a joining of the client's and our energy fields, a complete connection of mutual being.

4. Place your hands on either side of the head without touching. What is your immediate sense of the person? Is there a reaction inside of your body? You and your client have become one energetically. What is your body, your energy field, telling you in reaction to this mergence? What does it feel like? Is it peaceful? Chaotic? Do you feel trauma? Maybe something you can't yet

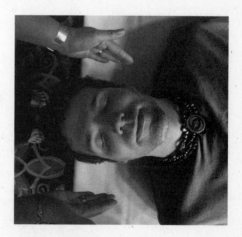

identify? That is okay. Don't spend a lot of time thinking about it. The client's system will reveal everything as you move through it. Remember, it is always best to go with your first impressions.

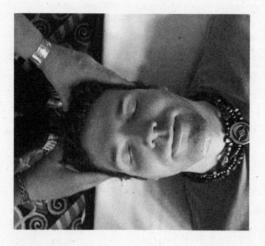

5. Next, place your thumbs directly on the subject's crown and let your hands lay gently along the side of the head and face. Use your body as a gyroscope. Is the centerline, the pranic tube, where it should be? Is it off center? Is it at a diagonal? Is there motion in the field that moves? Remember your commands here are:

- **ALIGN**

- **CENTER**

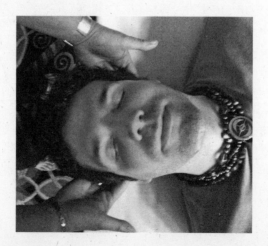

6. Next, touch the occipital "bumps" on the base of the skull with your hands under the head and your fingertips resting on the occipital bones. Is there balance here? Movement? What is your sense?

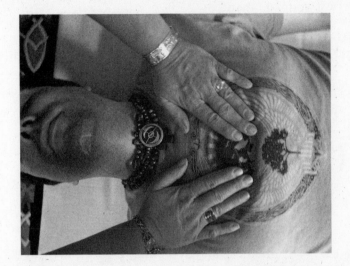

7. Place your hands at angles on the upper chest with fingers toward the centerline. This area will feel very different than the others you have touched so far. What is your sense here? Are both sides equal? Is one warmer or more intense than the other? If they are not the same, your command is:

- EQUALIZE (or)

- BALANCE

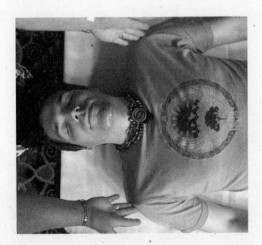

8. Slide your hands gently across the chest to the shoulders. Place your fingertips on the outside of the shoulders. Is there balance here? What is your sense? Often this area will feel as if one side is higher than the other. If this is the case, your command is:

   ⊛ **BALANCE**

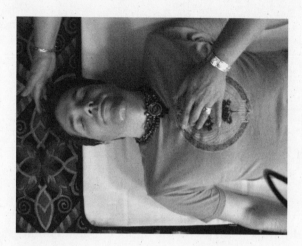

9. There are no commands needed for 8 through 12. The connections you make automatically create harmonization. Move around to the side of the body. Place the tips of your fingers of one hand on the crown, the fingertips of the other hand, just below the throat. Your command here is: HARMONIZE. Wait for a shift. It will be very subtle and usually takes just a few seconds.

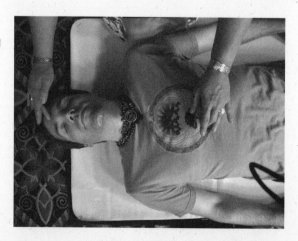

10. Move your upper hand down to the third eye area. In the same manner as you just touched the crown and throat areas, now touch the third eye and heart. Your command here is: HARMONIZE Wait for a shift. Once you have felt a change, it is okay to move to the next position.

11. Move down to the throat area. Touch the throat and solar plexus. Your command here is: HARMONIZE Wait for the shift. Once you have felt it, move to the next step.

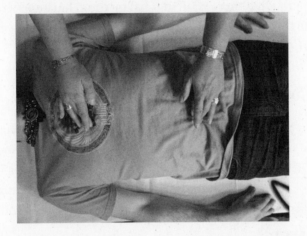

12. Move down to the heart area. Touch the heart and second chakra. Your command here is: HARMONIZE Wait for the shift. Once you have felt it, move to the next step.

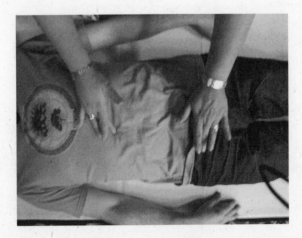

13. Move down to the solar plexus area. Touch the solar plexus and root chakra. Your command here is: HARMONIZE (When working around the root chakra, always be mindful about where exactly you put your hands!) Wait for the shift. Once you have felt it, move to the next step.

14. At any time when you touch the chakras in this way, you are creating a harmonic resonance among these areas. You may be guided to touch between the knees or ankles, or to lay an arm across the thighs. This is simply saying that there is further balance and harmonization needed as you make these corrections. Follow your instincts and *never, ever*, think about it. *Just do it.*

Checking the System's Balance

15. After you have completed harmonizing the alternating chakras, place one hand just below the throat area and one hand on the second chakra area. Do you feel the same sensation in both places? Is one area warm and the other cool? Both cool? Both warm and even? One more intense than the other? If so, keep this in mind for later. Sometimes using the command:

     ◦ BALANCE

     will correct the imbalance but not usually. The balance here will come later after you have made corrections on all the other levels.

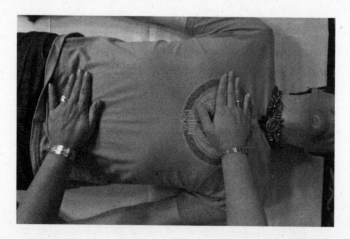

16. Leave the one hand on the second chakra, remove the other hand from the throat area, and place it on the crown. Remember to center your palm. Assess whether there is balance and equality of these two places. Again, this is a balance point and one that knows what to do when you connect the two places.

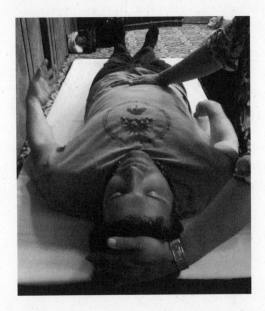

17. Next, touch the upper arm and the outside center of the calf simultaneously. Is there balance here? If not, wait until there is a shift and both places feel the same. There is no command needed here. The field will respond to the connection you are making.

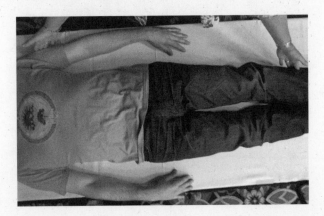

18. Move around to the knee area now. Place your thumbs on the inside of the knee and two or three of your fingers on the outside of the knee. What do you feel? Are you given any messages here? (Remember that often past life or other info may come to you here. If it does, whatever it is, it is important to the current life experience of your subject.) Your commands here are:

- **BALANCE**

- **ALIGN**

- **EQUALIZE**

19. Place your fingers on the outside of the anklebone, your thumbs on the center top of the foot. Are both sides even? Does one side feel higher or longer than the other? Is everything centered? Your commands here are:

- **ALIGN or STRAIGHTEN**

- **BALANCE**

- **EQUALIZE**

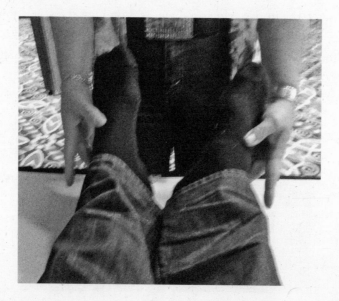

20. Let your fingers slide up the outside of the feet, and place the outside edge
of your little fingers in the crook where the little toe joins the foot. Be still
and wait for the shift. You may find yourself rocking back and forth, side
to side, or forward and backward. If you are, you are simply riding the
current of your subject's energy. As you make changes with the foot positions of your hands, you may notice that the energy is changing direction.
Optimally, you will want it to flow straight in alignment with the body so
that you are swaying straight in alignment with the subject as he lies on the
table. These connections require no commands.

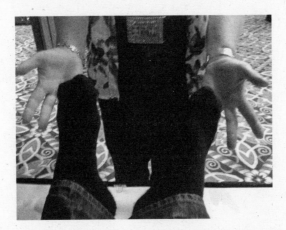

21. Place your thumbs on the tops of the big toes with your fingertips spread
and pointed outward, away from the body. Wait for the shift.

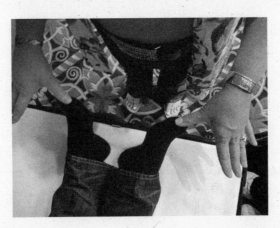

Level Two: Working with the Chakra System

Level two takes the practitioner through specific and overall balancing of the chakra system. An aware healer can utilize her intuitive nature to learn a great deal about the client as the chakras are accessed and worked with. Working the chakras should be done slowly and deliberately as the more fully the healer becomes immersed in the chakras, the more they will reveal.

After removal of any foreign debris, the basic commands for the chakras are:

- **DISSIPATE**: For blockages or inflammation.

- **CALIBRATE**: To correct length or direction of spin.

- **ASSIMILATE**: For bringing together fragmented pieces of the vortex that are usually only found in the throat and/or solar plexus but may occasionally be found elsewhere.

- **ALIGN**: To correct positioning.

- **CLARIFY**: To remove debris from the inside of the vortex.

- **REPAIR**: For torn chakra walls, particularly the second chakra.

- **ATTUNE**: To correct harmonics. This command should ALWAYS be the last correction you make because if you attune and haven't corrected anything else yet, the attunement won't remain.

When working with the chakras, use only one hand. Touch the chakra area with one or more fingers or with a flat palm or with the back of the hand. Your other hand should be away from the body. You may notice that your free hand moves into different mudra positions as you move from chakra to chakra. This is normal. Don't think about what your hand is doing. It is naturally seeking the best energy balance for the current connection between you and your subject. This is demonstrated in the pictures accompanying each chakra position. The pictures that follow are simply examples. There is no right or wrong mudra for the respective chakra positions.

1. Return to the head, and place your thumbs on the crown as you did at the beginning of the session, allowing your hands to rest alongside the face and head. Remember that each time you return to the head it may feel somewhat different. Feel for balance. When you feel "solid" with your touch there, move on to adjusting the chakras.

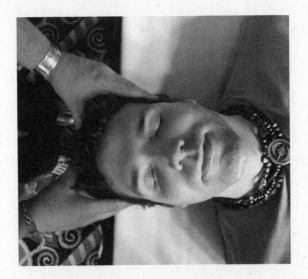

2. **Crown**—The energy here should be white. You can use a fingertip to instigate a spiral pattern in the flow of energy. A little tickle of the crown in a clockwise manner will coax it up for you if you aren't feeling it yet.

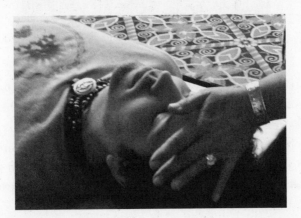

Next, place your palm centered directly onto the crown chakra. What is the feeling of the vortex here? Is it elongated, compacted, straight, bent, just right? The vortex should flow clockwise. Whatever you feel, if it is out of normal, command change until you see or feel the shift. After you have found balance, polarity, and frequency, slowly raise your palm out from the crown, and as you do so, imagine that the pyramid here gains perfect clarity, size, and height. This field should be clear and white.

3. **The third eye** is often off center and can be, but is rarely, fragmented. It is indigo in color. There may be blockages in this area. Sometimes it rises up above the forehead and to one side or the other. Usually if it has moved to one side, it has gone to the left but not always. Clear the blockages first and then command the vortex/pyramid back to center. Next, check the color frequencies and command any change that is necessary.

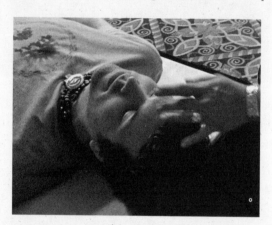

4. **The throat chakra** is an icy blue and is often fragmented, matrixed, off center, or has affectations or junk energy that has collected there. The order of repair is remove affectations (any foreign or junk energy) first, separate the matrixing, assimilate the fragments to center, and center the field. This area has to do with issues of trust, control, loneliness, and whether or not one has felt free to speak one's truth. There is a direct relationship with the second chakra.

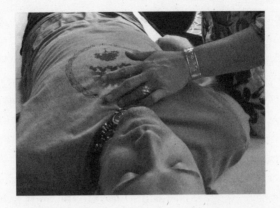

5. **Heart chakra area**—This area should be a bright, clear Kelly green. Most common issues are belief conflicts, self-protection, and a lack of understanding one's personal truth. This area will most commonly become withdrawn, reversed, shallow, and spread across the chest, diffuse (weak in charge), fragmented, blocked, or a combination of several of these things. This area will often give one a sense of historic issues. Order of repair: Remove any affectations found, extract if withdrawn (sunken into the body), assimilate the energies into a single vortex if necessary, clear blockages, begin appropriate rotation pattern, correct the frequencies.

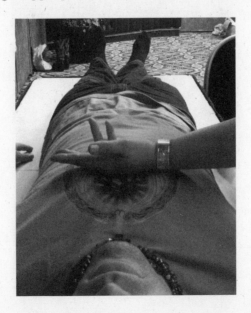

6. **Solar plexus**—This area is a sunny yellow when normal. The solar plexus area has to do with one's self-expression, relationships, and creativity. There is often energy of underlying anger that has caused issues here. There are also often blockages here. Remember that this is the exchange point between the above and the below energies and that this field is vital to the health of the organs and overall energetic system. Affectations may be found here, as this is also where one takes on the energies of others. There might be junk energy collecting here, or may be matrixing (usually), fragmentation, a reversal of the vortex, withdrawal, or other affectations. This vortex often reverses polarity and sinks into the body in a self-defensive posturing. Remember, always remove foreign affectations first, then the matrixing repair, assimilation, centering, blockages, repair inflamed energies, and then fine tune the vortex.

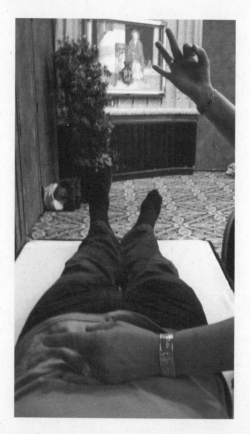

7. **The second chakra** is a brightly lit orange when normal. It has to do with one's sense of personal validation or value. It is also how we feel that others see us. Often there is interruption of the spin due to affectations taken on by a dominant person in childhood, when their values did not feel true. Always remove the affectation first. Very often there is resistance to repairs in the second chakra area. If you find this to be true, patiently wait for the necessary changes to occur. If there is still resistance, ask your subject to breathe into your hand as it rests on the chakra. There may be a thickening of the outside of the vortex, protection or scarring due to affectations. This must be changed to normal free spinning energy of a clockwise direction. This area often needs to be attuned to normal frequencies. There may be a self-protective withdrawing of this field into the body as well.

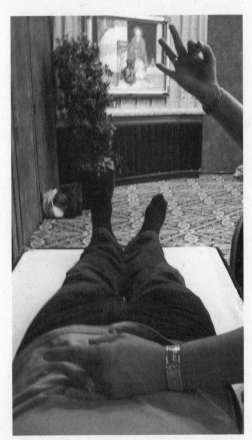

8. **First chakra**—This area is a deep red when normal. It is most often under-charged or tilted or too deep on plane, slightly sunken into the body. If needed, straighten the vortex, replanting it solidly upon the centerline and then charging it to normal frequencies.

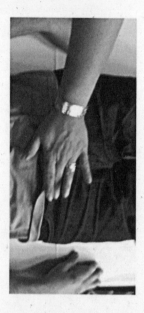

9. Repeat the balance check process: After you have completed harmonizing the chakras, place one hand just below the throat area and one hand on the second chakra area. Do you feel the same sensation in both places? Is one area warm and the other cool? Both cool? Both warm and even? One more intense than the other? If so, keep this in mind for later. Sometimes using the command:

   • **BALANCE**

   will correct the imbalance but not usually. The balance here will come later after you have made corrections on all the other levels.

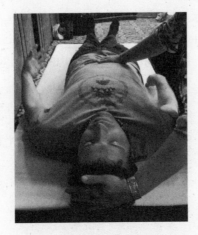

10. Leave the one hand on the second chakra, remove the other hand from the throat area, and place it on the crown. Remember to center your palm. Assess whether there is balance and equality of these two places. Again, this is a balance point and one that knows what to do when you connect the two places.

11. Next, touch the upper arm and the outside center of the calf simultaneously. Is there balance here? If not, wait until there is a shift and both places feel the same. There is no command needed here. The field will respond to the connection you are making.

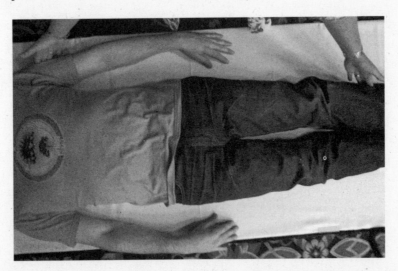

Move around to the feet area now. Place your thumbs on the inside of the feet and lay your hands over the top of the feet. Let your fingers fall naturally. What do you feel? Are you given any messages here?

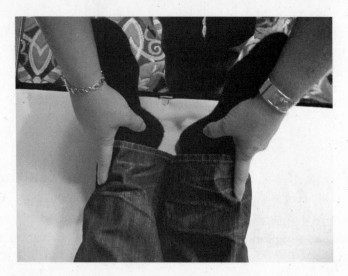

Finally, with your thumb and finger, grasp the soft spot next to the base of the big toe and the bottom of the foot in the corresponding spot. What do you feel here? Do the two sides feel equal? Of so great. If not, the key word here is BALANCE.

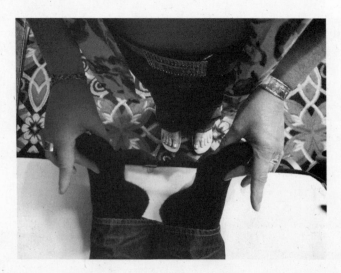

Level Three: Working with the Etheric and Physical Bodies

Level three is exquisitely powerful and is very likely to cause the client to leave her body temporarily. It is vital to watch her particularly through this phase to make sure she is breathing at all times. When a person leaves her body, she often begin to breathe with what seems to be a light snore, but the breathing is shallow and slow. This is ultimate relaxation.

It is also an extremely blissful experience, and some clients don't want to come back because it feels so good or they have become unaware of the practitioner or anything else in the third dimension. Great care must be taken to gently rouse the client at the end of the session. Maintaining physical touch during the session is very helpful to assist a person back to her body.

The Etheric bodies have three kinds of alignment: On center (even in line with the other bodies except the causal bodies which are either side of the stack), On plane (should lie parallel to the other bodies and flat, not angled up or down) and on parallel (sometimes a body slides out of position away from the stack of other bodies. This one is particularly related to the causal bodies).

After removing any foreign debris, your commands for the Etheric bodies are:

- **ALIGN**: To correct positioning in relation to the other bodies

- **DISSIPATE**: To remove blockages or inflammation

- **CLARIFY**: To unify the harmonics in the body

- **CALIBRATE**: Corrects size and density of the body

- **REPAIR**: Fixes tears and holes in the body's walls

- **ATTUNE**: Corrects harmonics of the bodies in relation to the entire system

First, with your hands palms up and over the body, ask the bodies to RISE and DISPLAY. When you do, the bodies will separate and rise above the physical body so that you can access them.

1. **Emotional Body**—Can be small or too large, swollen, mottled in color, off color, corded to the physical or the mental, blocked, off center with the

other bodies, or contain foreign affectations. The energy of this body may be confused or entangled with the energies of the mental body in a person who is really "in their head" all the time.

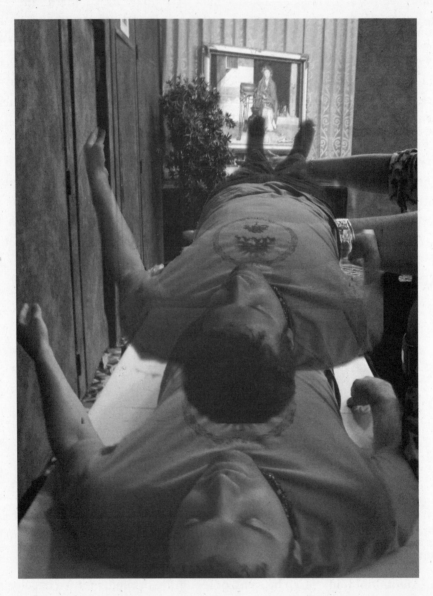

2. **Mental**—Is bright yellow. May be corded by emotional, usually shows inflammations of energy in certain areas. These are generally specific and can be identified as relative to the underlying issues by the location of the dysfunction.

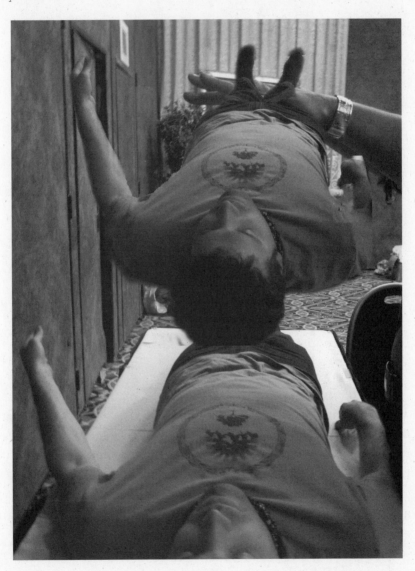

3. **Intuitive**—Is white with a violet or purple mantle over the shoulders. This body is generally normal but may show affectations of being over large, small, or off center. Blockages in this field are rare but do occur.

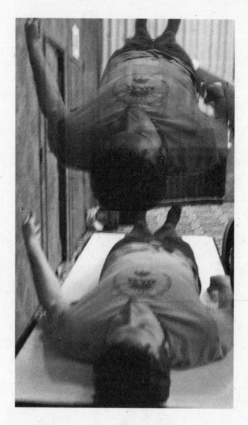

4. **The Causal Bodies:** The Causal bodies are varying in color, and range from mottled greens and browns to mottled teals, greens, and blues. These bodies are the Octave point harmonically. They may display giftedness in a person. If these bodies are carrying anything unusual, these things are generally related to those gifts and should not be removed. These bodies are out to the sides from center in good balance. They are the most ancient aspects of manifestation in the journey of the soul. Usually the only repairs needed here are of tattering around the edges of the bodies as they have had long and difficult passages. These bodies are a source of strength and balance. Affectations other than those already mentioned are extremely

rare but do occur. Those found in this area such as blockages or injuries have been present for most of the incarnations and often are found in chronic pain or other serious illness or pain. They can be repaired.

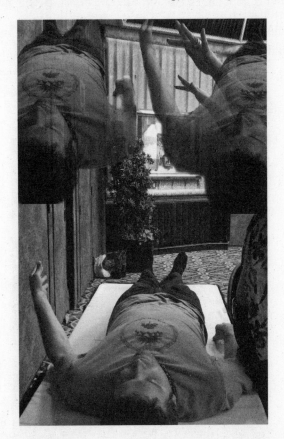

5. **The Soul**—The body of the soul is pure white and is almost always perfect. I may have seen one that had a necessary repair in all these years! It is the area surrounding that will show issues, blockages, etc. Check the area around this body for blockages. Often the densities of the blockage are tiny here. Large ones or ones that are intense feeling are usually current Karmic influences. We can clear the blockage so that the soul has a better ability to make choices in its journey, but we should never try to remove someone's Karma. Karma is part of the journey of the soul. On occasion we may find inactive densities that feel lighter but inert. These are older

blockages from old Karmic influences that no longer apply and we can clear those. For the area around the soul, your commands are:

- **DISSIPATE:** Blockages and old Karmic energies that are no longer active

- **CLARIFY:** Completely clears the field of any tiny impurities that dissipation did not clear

- **CALIBRATE:** Retunes the field density

- **ATTUNE:** Unifies the harmonics in this area

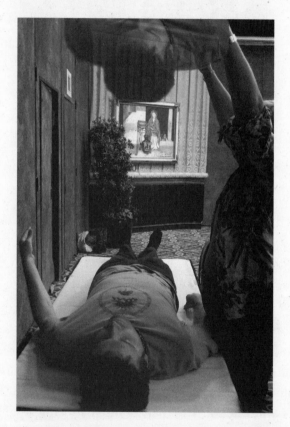

6. **Physical**—Scan the body with your senses or your hands for necessary changes and create those changes. Some areas will feel warmer or colder than others. A great rule of thumb here is that those areas that get your attention need your attention.

If you are uncertain of what you are feeling, don't imagine something just to have something to say. Do the best that you can to make the repairs that are needed and then be honest with your client if you have made changes and don't understand them. If you do get information, be sure to share this in a kind and loving way. Remember, this isn't about you, so you have no need to have an attachment to the outcome. Speak from your heart and gently. Sometimes it is best to speak of possibilities rather than certainties! Remember:

The physical body has many layers and areas of harmonics, so it is a good idea to scan the body with your hand and make corrections in local areas as they are found. Any or all of the following basic commands may apply:

- **ALIGN**: If meridian lines do not seem to be in alignment. They can move if the pranic tube was not centered or if the chakras were not functioning well.

- **DISSIPATE**: To remove blockages or inflammation anywhere in or on the body.

- **CLARIFY**: To unify the harmonics in an area such as in the organs.

- **CALIBRATE**: Corrects energy flow if you find an area that is running too much or too slow.

- **REPAIR**: Fixes tears and holes in the energy field.

- **ATTUNE**: Corrects harmonics pretty much anywhere.

7. After you have completed harmonizing the Etheric bodies, place one hand just below the throat area and one hand on the second chakra area. Do you feel the same sensation in both places? Is one area warm and the other cool? Both cool? Both warm and even? One more intense than the other? If so, keep this in mind for later. Sometimes using the command:

- **BALANCE**

will correct the imbalance but not usually. The balance here will come later after you have made corrections on all the other levels.

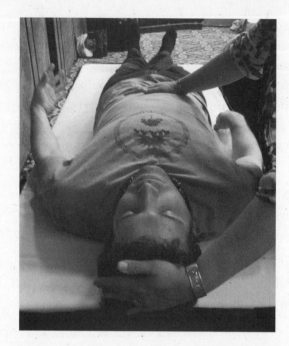

8. Leave the one hand on the second chakra, remove the other hand from the throat area, and place it on the crown. Remember to center your palm. Assess whether there is balance and equality of these two places. Again, this is a balance point and one that knows what to do when you connect the two places.

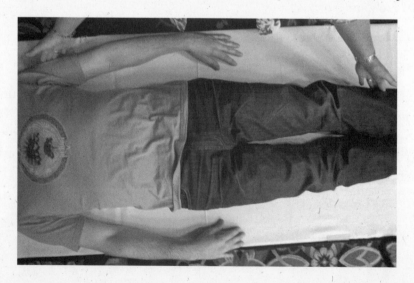

9. Next, touch the upper arm and the outside center of the calf simultane-
    ously. Is there balance here? If not, wait until there is a shift and both
    places feel the same. There is no command needed here. The field will
    respond to the connection you are making.

    Move around to the feet area now. Place your thumbs on the inside of the
    knees and two or three of your fingers on the outside of the knees. What do
    you feel? Are you given any messages here?

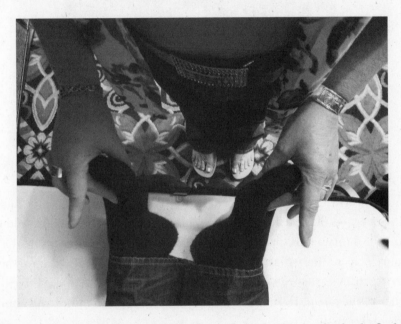

10. Step back from the body. Walk around the body slowly; look, feel, sense,
    if there is anything further to do. This is about fine-tuning what you
    have already done. Last minute items will likely get your attention. At
    times, even something major may show up once the system has been
    attuned and there is clearer access. If you are guided to adjust or change
    anything further, do so. Check the balances as described above one
    more time.

11. From the head, work your way around the exterior field and clear it of
    blockages and trash. Repair any other things that you find here (attach-
    ments, anomalies, tears).

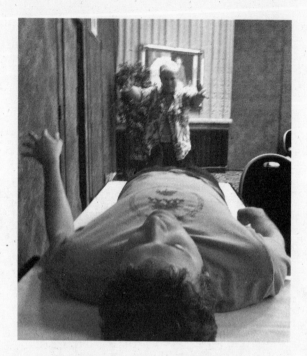

When working with the external field, we may find that it is misshapen. The energies may be flowing in all kinds of crazy patterns. The field walls may be damaged or torn, and there may be blockages present in one or more places. There may also be thought forms present that can present as living things that are symbolic of the angst they create in the life experience of the client. Here are the anomalies most often found and commands to correct them:

If the field is not a perfect elliptical shape or if the energies within it are not fluid, like water in a clear bag, command the field to:

• **CALIBRATE**

If the energy inside of this field is more than one color or colors that are not harmonic with each other (i.e., colors that don't match or go with each other), this means that the interior of the external field is disharmonic so we tell it to:

• **HARMONIZE**

If there is a tear in the outer wall:

* **REPAIR**

If there are blockages or dense areas of energy that are interfering with the fluidity of this energy field:

* **DISSIPATE**

After any and all repairs that are found are made:

* **ATTUNE**

12. Next, from the head area as well, check the axiom points. Remember that these are the grid connections. Make sure that all are functional. Make sure that each axiom point feels alive and active. Some may not feel as if they are lit up. A simple command to normalize will bring its charge back up. Your commands here are:

   * **BALANCE**: To adjust intensity of axiom point. Remember, they should all feel identical.

   * **LIGHT**: To re-ignite an axiom point that is not working.

   * **DISSIPATE**: Removes inflammation or overcharge of energy.

   * **DECOMPRESS**: Relieves dense areas so the energy can flow better.

   * **CLARIFY**: Equalizes the energy inside the field's walls.

   * **CALIBRATE**: Corrects densities or irregularities to interior field flow.

   * **ATTUNE**: Corrects harmonization of the field.

After you have completed all three levels of the session, repeat the balance checks again. Place one hand just below the throat area and one hand on the second chakra area. Do you feel the same sensation in both places? By now there should be perfect balance between these areas, and they should feel identical in temperature and intensity. If there remains any slight imbalance, use the command:

* **BALANCE**

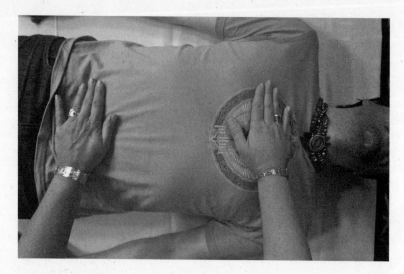

13. Leave the one hand on the second chakra, remove the other hand from
     the throat area, and place it on the crown. Remember to center your palm.
     Assess whether there is balance and equality of these two places. By now
     they should feel identical.

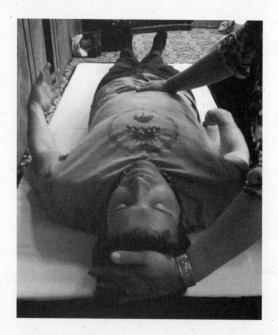

14. Next, touch the upper arm and the outside center of the calf simultane-
    ously. Is there balance here? Again, by now these places should feel identi-
    cal to each other. If not, wait until there is a shift and both places feel the
    same. There is no command needed here. The field will respond to the con-
    nection you are making.

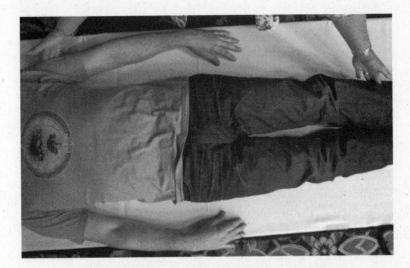

15. Move around to the feet area now. Place your thumbs on the inside of the
    feet and lay your hands over the top of the feet. Let your fingers fall natu-
    rally. What do you feel? Are you given any messages?

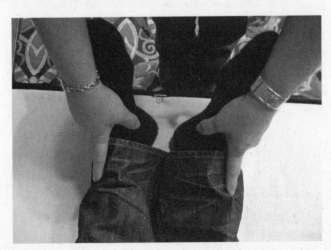

16. Once you are satisfied that all balance points are equal and there is nothing further to do, go down to the area of the feet. From the feet, step back and separate yourself from the field. Bring your hands together and intentionally and reverently close your connection with your subject. Do this with gratitude for having had the opportunity to assist them. Quietly express to the body honor for having been within its fields, and then step back away from the energy field.

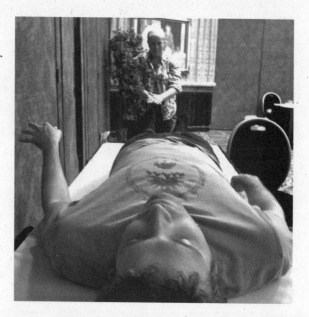

17. Allow your client to come back gently if he has drifted off or left his body. Watch to make certain that he continues to breathe regularly. If you need to approach him due to time constraints or otherwise, do so very gently by a light touch on the arm or leg; speak extremely softly. Repeat several times if necessary, and request him to return.

In NO WAY, NEVER, EVER, leave a person alone in a room after working with them, especially if they are "out" of their body. STAY WITH THEM at all times until they are COMPLETELY LUCID AND REGAIN COORDINATION.

CHAPTER ELEVEN

The Language of the Living Light: Using the Symbols after General Healing Session

The first time I saw the symbols of the living light was on the Master's robe in the pyramid chamber. Remember, he was the first Master to step into me to teach me from the inside out. The experience was so powerful that I actually didn't remember seeing the symbols at first. Only later, as the symbols became part of me, did I remember when and where they had first graced my presence.

As I became more enlightened, more aware, the symbols began to appear in my visions. Usually, when they first came only one would reveal itself. Then another, then another, until whole pages of the symbols ran through my vision. I began writing them down, attempting to re-create them in my own clumsy way.

The symbols are living light. Light that is organized in the form of glyphs. Not only are they beautiful, they have great purpose. Each one of the symbols is a full library of teachings, of memory that is stored in the ethers.

My access to the symbols came after I projected my consciousness through an Etheric gateway. It was in the form of a rectangle that floated out in front of me, beckoning me to enter. As I projected my consciousness through the doorway, I found myself being propelled toward a bright star far in the distance. I was moving so fast I couldn't make out any details except my destination.

Later after my return from that journey, the symbols began to command my attention, taking over my reality at times. They seemed to come out of nowhere, filling my sight and my mind. I had no idea how to interpret them, and so as I had done everything else, I just let them free flow in my awareness.

I knew that the symbols were powerful forms of information and attunement for me, but I didn't really have a clue as to what practical use they had. After a time, they began to appear while I was performing healing sessions. I began to see them on people's bodies, and as I became more experienced with them, I also realized that the symbols had specific places on and over the bodies of my clients.

I began to draw the symbols with my fingers. It wasn't like I meant to; it just happened. As I fluidly moved through the energy fields of my clients, placing symbols became a natural part of the process. It seemed like the more I used the symbols, the more would come until I began to see them raining down on my clients.

As they fell, the symbols changed color, undulated, and turned in a free fall. As they came, the energy in my body responded. I felt strangely light and as if my entire energy field had unified to meet them and I had become the doorway for them to enter.

Even later, my fingers began to move independently of each other, each drawing different symbols and all drawing at once. If I thought about it, my fingers could not intentionally repeat the movement, but when I just let them go, the symbols flowed out of my fingers and all over the bodies of my clients. Sometimes there were so many I couldn't comprehend them.

I had heard about Reiki, and that it works using specific symbols, but these experiences were not as specific. It looked and felt as if I had opened a cosmic floodway and the symbols were cascading out, raining around me, through me, even at times of me. I began to notice that when I used them, specific areas of energy changed in an instant. They could be used to transmute energy to different frequencies. They could be placed to seal repairs that I had made to the energy system. They could also be used to "teach" an energy field to create the realities that my clients requested. Honestly, it was mind-blowing watching the symbols free flow through the air and then into place. They automatically knew where to place themselves.

As I began to share the symbols individually with my clients and then, later, groups of people, I further realized that each individual symbol, when experienced by a person, was an energetic initiation. When people held them or looked at them, something happened in their energy fields. The symbols were attuning their energy fields to higher frequencies, literally changing the vibration.

I began to insert symbols and combinations of them into my newsletters, the Online Messages, and soon realized that my readers were printing them out, taping them virtually everywhere in their homes on their refrigerators, their mirrors, in their cars, at work, everywhere. My readers told me that there was something familiar about them that they just couldn't place but something . . .

And they feel so good.

As time went on, I began to learn the placement patterns of specific symbols, and I began to instruct my students about when and where to place them. As my students used them, I could feel the energy in the room shift and change frequencies. I could see the energy fields of my students changing frequencies. They could feel it. And soon, different layers of symbols began to present themselves, as if each layer had specific applications and purpose.

Each layer of symbols is a specific attunement on multi-dimensional levels of reality as well as within the physical body. The direction in which the symbol is placed changes its frequencies as well as its meaning.

The names of the symbols are not really pronounceable because they are combinations of frequencies and not words. Words define too completely and the symbols are alive, changing meaning, color, sound, and frequencies.

Included here are several layouts of how the symbols are placed. They can be used in the overall healing process that you are learning in this book, or they can be utilized as a process all their own. They must be laid down in a specific order because, as they are, fields of harmonics are being created. To lay down the symbols out of order would be to temporarily create a disharmony that has a completely different reality than the correct order. When given in the wrong order, the symbols create a completely different set of harmonics that can be damaging to the fine balance of an energy system.

Remember, the symbols are individual sets of living harmonics. They are complete libraries of information, and when combined, the reality of their messages changes. As they are used in a specific order, the symbols harmonize together to create a specific reality. When they are rearranged, a different reality occurs harmonically so order is extremely important!

Applying the Symbols

Quick reprogramming and universal harmony can be brought to a subtle energy system by drawing the symbols upon the body in the order shown in the following diagram. It is important to remember that the symbols on the cards are entire libraries of information that will be conveyed, so no extra information or intention needs to be provided for this exercise.

The symbols work quickly, harmonizing with each other as they are laid out, but once the last symbol is set out, it is a great idea to give the recipient about fifteen minutes to let the harmonization fully set in. It is most advisable to use the symbols sets in the order listed below. Each set can be used as a singular treatment, but these are based upon holographic and multi-dimensional reality, so each set of symbols builds first on itself, as the symbols are laid out, and then in harmonic resonance with the other sets of symbols as they are added. The ideal way to use these is after the basic session is completed and all corrections and repairs that were needed in the Etheric anatomy have been accomplished. Then the harmonics of the symbols sets will calibrate into the system more easily and fully. The symbols sets are meant to instill not only a full harmonization but also a cosmic education that is coded onto the particulates and DNA of the subject who is receiving them.

Here is how they work:

Level One: The Light Body (Soul) Attunement in Conjunction with the Physical, or Earthly, Being

When this body is out of balance, you may have forgotten your freedom as a soul who has traveled from lifetime to lifetime, creating opportunities to feel, to love, to learn, to experience everything that is tactile and that which is intangible. Your only limitation is the belief that you are merely physical. In your dreams as a child you flew, and then you fell as you began to believe that flying was impossible and that the physical was all you were. That was when untruth became your reality. You can fly without falling any time you are ready.

This body is your true self, unlimited by mass or density, free of boundaries and limitations. It is the body with which you travel in your dreams and that has filled your physical being with the very life that you live. When harmonized and balanced, this body reflects your original set of harmonics, and you begin to work as a strong and unified set of energy combined directly with the light of the source. Once re-harmonized in this body, you are at a pinnacle of your existence, ready to fly beyond the known. All it takes to change the direction of your journey from this moment forward is a leap of faith.

In order to proceed with the living light attunement, place symbols in the following order:

1. The crown

2. The third eye

3. The throat

4. The heart

5. The solar plexus

6. The Second Chakra

7. The First Chakra

8. The high heart (just above and to the left of center chest)

9. The body center (Dan Jun) (just above the second chakra)

10. Right upper shoulder

11. Left upper shoulder

12. Right hip

13. Left hip

14. Right hand

15. Left hand

16. Right knee

17. Left knee

18. Right foot

19. Left foot

The full set of symbols for this body looks like this:

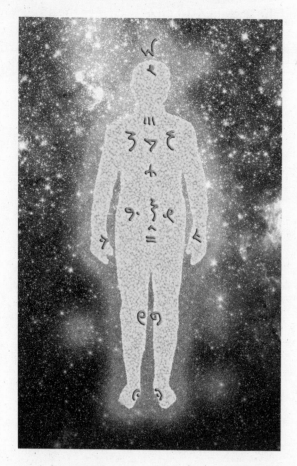

Harmonizing the Body (Back Side)

Further fine-tuning harmonization can be added to the backside of the body if you wish. Draw the symbols in the order below as per the picture. Give the person another fifteen minutes to experience the symbols before removing them.

1. The body history (goes above the head)

2. The body mid-back (center of upper back)

3. The body small of back (just above the sacrum)

4. The kidneys (one over each kidney right first, then left side)

5. The wing points (place just to the inside of the scapula)

6. In this now (away from the body, above and diagonal from right shoulder)

7. The quiet within (away from the body across from right side mid-calf)

8. As it has always been (away from the body across from the left mid-calf)

9. Harmony (away from the body above and diagonal from the left shoulder)

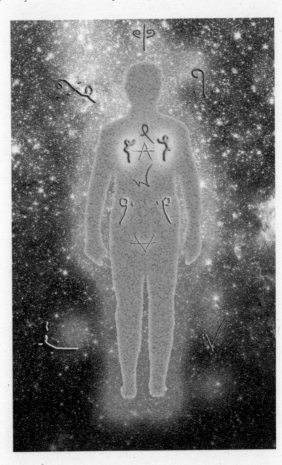

Level Two: The Body Galactic—Attunement to Our Universal Balance

There are parts of us that live simultaneously in the past, present, and future. They exist outside of time and space. They are enthusiastic travelers into the unknown, willing participants in experience and knowledge of all kinds. When we are in balance, our Galactic body is working in every glint of a moment to bring us infinite awareness of worlds beyond our comprehension.

Place the symbols in the following order:

1. Spiral over heart area

2. Crown

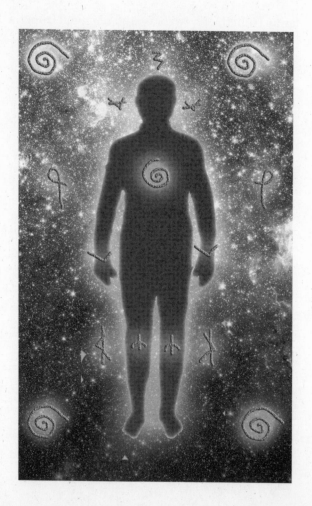

3. Left hand

4. Right hand

5. Left knee

6. Right knee

7. Either side of head, left side, then right side

8. Either side of knees, left side, then right side

9. Away from body, upper arm, left side, then right side

10. Spiral upper left

11. Spiral lower left

12. Spiral lower right

13. Spiral upper right

Level Three: The Body Unified—Locking Multi-Level Attunements in Place

When we have not locked in our balance across dimensions, we have not yet truly considered, or allowed, that the balance of body, mind, and spirit are connected infinitely in our experience as a soul. We seek our divinity as if it were a separate aspect, or an accomplishment to be attained. Out of harmony, we often struggle with our body, our thoughts, or our spiritual nature, believing that one or the other or all need to be healed. We must look again. We are inherently perfect. All else is perception.

This set of symbols represents the marriage of our humanity with our divinity. When we have found balance with all of our aspects, including both our human and divine selves, we operate as One with creation. We are divine in our humanness. When these symbols are placed, we harmonize and energize our energy field as human beings with all of our physical as well as our multi-dimensional energy fields and we lock in the balance.

We are eternally harmonized and open to a continuous flow of information and energy.

Apply these symbols as follows:

1. Heart

2. Root

3. Left side

4. Right side

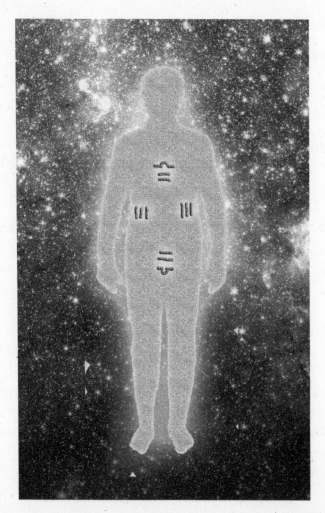

Level Four: Attuning the Ascension Body (Codes the DNA and Attunes All Levels of the Etheric Anatomy to Ascension Level of Gamma Consciousness)

Perhaps our mind believes in Ascension, but our heart has not connected with the fact that we are beings of the light. We shouldn't resist in separateness but instead work from within the One, not at it. By allowing ourselves to become immersed beyond our thinking mind and into unlimited consciousness, we can find freedom beyond our imaginings.

When the body, mind, and spirit come into full balance and we are free enough to access our ability to reach into higher levels of consciousness, certain changes occur in our bodies. The higher consciousness expands our subtle energy field and that, in turn, speaks to our DNA, which also expands. As this occurs, there comes a moment of unification of all our energy fields that shifts us into ascension mode. From there, we can return into the infinite at will.

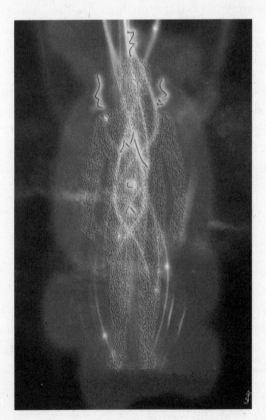

To attune the ascension body, place the symbols in the following order:

1. Crown

2. Heart

3. Solar plexus

4. Second Chakra

5. Above left shoulder

6. Above right shoulder

Long Distance Healing

All of the principles and methods that we have used so far can also be applied to long distance healing. In the same way that we merge with the energy field of another person when she is present, we can travel outside of time and space to join her ethereally.

Not only is consciousness superluminal, faster than the speed of light, it is also not restricted to boundaries that apply to time and space. In order to connect with someone ethereally, all we need to do is send our consciousness out into the ethers. In the same way that energy knows where to go when it is directed by intention, so does our consciousness. It will go straight to where it is intended by recognizing the frequencies of our target subject. Once our consciousness has located our target, it immediately merges with them as we intended.

Once we have established a mergence with our subject, we can go through the healing process as if he were in the same room with us. When I first began to do long distance work, I went to my healing room and actually worked at my healing table as if the person were there with me. Much to my delight, I was able to feel their energy fields with my hands and to see them as well. Later, as I became more proficient with long distance healing, I didn't need to go through the motions any longer and was able to sit comfortably almost anywhere and move into a safe mergence with my clients and do the work.

Sample Long Distance Sessions

I began to transcribe the sessions as I did them so that I could send a detailed record to my clients. They really appreciate having these, and I highly suggest providing a transcript whenever possible. A typical session looks like this:

Session (Anonymous)
OCTOBER 2007
Access is granted.

We are requested to assess and work with issues, if given, of general opening and personal freedom as well as assisting in repair of an injury of the low back.

Our first impression is of a generally blocked external energy field. There is no fluidity and little freedom of movement in general of the external energy system. There is physical trauma here and emotional trauma as well. We clarify this field and find that once the overall blockage is removed there is fragmentation most likely due to physical trauma. We also find that there are leakages within the exterior field that would be causal to a slowing of physical energy.

We assimilate the fragmentation into one functional unit. Next, we repair leakages, which are extensive. We continue clarification of the field until it is of perfect fluidity. It is done.

The area of the crown is elongated and unstable. This being is of a mental nature, perhaps if only of late. There has been much worry and concern within this being. We recalibrate this vortex to perfection of length and density. Next, we attune for perfection of frequencies. It is done.

The area of the third eye is off center and elongated. This is an unusual formation. We relocate the vortex to exact center and root it there. We calibrate to perfection.

The area of the throat is greatly fragmented. This area is representative of physical trauma, emotional trauma, trust, control, and one's feelings of safety to speak his inner truth. We assimilate the fragmentation and attune to proper frequency and functioning. There is a moderate energy leakage here, which we repair.

The area of the heart vortex is blocked with dense energy patterns. There is self-protection here. We transmute the blockage to find that this is a sensitive being who always strives to do what is right from his heart perspective. We continue to clarify until clear. Next, we assimilate the heart energies to perfection of harmonic relations. It is done.

The area of the solar plexus is greatly matrixed and fragmented. There is energetic debris here. This area is related to issues of relationship, creativity, and self-expression. It is where the energies of the above and the below are exchanged. This area also feeds the organs energetically and is directly related to the mid-back. We clarify the debris from the field and transmute it to normal light energy. We separate the matrixing and align along normal meridian pathways. We assimilate the fragmentation into one functional unit of energy. Next, we reduce inflammation and remove blockage. We root at exact center and plane to perfection of harmonic relationships.

The area of the second vortex is fragmented into three distinct aspects. We assimilate this. Next, we find that polarity is reversed and correct this. This area has to do with issues of how one sees himself and how he feels others see him. He continues to see himself as broken rather than the perfect being that he is. When he is able to remember his inner perfection, he will begin to heal more expediently and completely.

The area of the first vortex is withdrawn (self-protection) and in need of recharging. We correct placement and root at exact center and plane. Next we attune to perfection.

The emotional body displays several energy leaks. We repair these. The body is swollen in self-protection. We calibrate to normal density and size. Next, we clarify the body of injuries and attune to perfection of harmonic resonance.

The mental body is blocked about the trunk. There has been much mental cycling, perhaps concern or worry, or attempts to understand something which is greater than the mind can perceive.

One wonders why he has had the recent experience of injury. If he were to look honestly at his life before the injury, he would find that he did not sit still long enough to really know how he felt, what his experience was. He looked ahead of himself and not in the moment. In such a way, he lost touch with some of his inner guidance and knowing. He operated more from a mental standpoint and so now realizes that there is more that his life has to offer him. He seeks the *perfection he does not see in himself, yet this is who he is. A perfect being of Creation. We clarify this body of all blockage and find that below the blockage was inflammation. We dissipate this.*

The intuitive body is angulated 170 degrees. We right the body and correct plane and placement.

The causal bodies are misaligned. We correct this.

The soul body is perfect as it would be. The area around this body indicates many Karmic situations in play in this now. We are given that this is mostly related to other people. That many of his current relationships are relative to solving challenges of his journey. If he recognizes patterns within his journey, he can simply choose differently than he has in the past, and in such a way, this will change the direction of the journey gently, for the most part and finalize the Karmic instances.

The physicality appears to be of generally good condition except that it is low in energy. Having repaired the energy leakages will assist in higher levels of vitality.

We are specifically requested to assist with issues of injury to the low back. It appears that the area of L3, L4 is of injury with misalignment of the spine as a result. This continues to exert pressure on the vertebrae, which is causal to impingement of the disk there. There is also pressure at L2.

From a metaphysical perspective, this area has to do with issues of responsibility. If this being would resolve his issues revolving around responsibility, there will come relief on an emotional level as well as physical healing. There is also within the tissues here, the belief that one is broken. He must, as we have said, find his perfection from the inside out. When he recognizes his perfection and sees himself as healed and healing, he will begin to have different life experience altogether, that of a positive nature. There continues to be inflammation of the tissues in the area. We instigate frequencies of 00273, 04975, 00797, 005097, aa273 and a4792. We fill the area with the harmonics and the request to normalize. There is movement of the vertebrae. We continue to bathe the area in these frequencies. Next, we add bb2798. Upon addition of this frequency we are given that the inflammation normalizes.

End of session.

As you can see, the long distance session is quite comprehensive and complete. After receiving this session, this person's life was completely changed. The pain went away and a complete change in life direction was made.

Here is another example:

Session (Anonymous)
June 2010
Access is granted.

We are requested to assist with issues of the following:

- *Anxiety issues*

- *My concerns are my weight and my fears. To be a little more specific, weight has always been my issue—battled with it all my life. I have been terrified to go to the doctor. My blood pressure shoots up and I am afraid the doctor is going to say I am dying.*

- *I am crazy about animals and have always had many dogs at one time. I am down to one dog and will not get another because I get so fearful every time the least little thing happens to them. I am so tied up in the health of myself and everyone around me—especially the dogs. I have started clenching my teeth and of course that leads to other issues—like TMJ.*

- *My mother tells me that when she was in labor with me, my dad was out of town and she refused to push to allow the baby to be born. The doctor kept telling her she had to let go and push, but she refused. I guess the doctor finally had to hit her over the head or something to release this baby—me. Perhaps this has to do with my fears, but I hate living like this.*

Our first impression is one of chaos in the external field. There are emotional issues at play which have been hidden in the field over this lifetime and have become errant in patterning in relation to the balance of the system. These are causal to anxiety and non-logical fear. The source comes from an incorrect assumption that she was unwanted at birth. Having these feelings leaves her anxious and fearful that she is not in control of anything in her life. She fears loss because she believed she was lost. The weight gain is protective and would dissipate once she realizes her value and her perfection. She fears to love, as in her dogs, for fear of losing. She fears death because she does not embrace life. She must begin to take steps to embrace her power in such a way that the empowerment overrides her fears and the fears are no longer the prevailing power.

We calibrate the external body to correction of patterning and liquidity. Next we attune to uniformity and attune for correction of frequency sets.

The crown vortex is inverted and angulated 11 degrees southeast. We correct polarity reversal and position of the vortex, correcting angulation simultaneously. Next we root the vortex at exact center and plane and calibrate for correction of length and density. One tends to look outside of herself for validation. She would be well served to trust her own values and self, for it is there that perfection and truth lie. We attune the vortex to perfection of harmonic resonance.

The third eye vortex is off plane and to the left. It is unattached and non-communicative with the system. We correct placement and root the vortex at exact center and plane and attune to highest possible resonance.

The throat vortex is fragmented and inverted deep into the body. This area is relative to issues of trust, control, trauma, and one's feelings of safety to speak her inner truth. This being has applied her trauma into a state of self-protection that has become self-consciousness and anxiety-ridden. We assimilate the fragmentation into the main vortex and extract it from the body. We clarify the vortex and repair the underlying field. Next we root the vortex into exact position on plane and center and calibrate it for correction of length and density. In these areas of being the subject also looks outward for validation that she does not receive. We further attune the vortex to perfection of harmonic resonance and clarify the area of dense blockages.

The heart vortex is inverted and widespread across the chest. This creates a drain of energy and therefore resources from the body. This is indicative of emotional self-protection, of living on the surface so that deeper feelings are not revealed and one's vulnerabilities are not betrayed. She would realize that what does not get in also does not get out. This contributes to the build-up of anxiety in the body. We assimilate the vortex energy and instigate oscillation of a newly formed vortex. Next, we calibrate the vortex for size and density and root it at exact center and plane. We repair the underlying field and decompress several moderate blockages in the chest area. Next we attune the vortex to perfection of harmonic resonance.

The solar plexus is also inverted and drawn inward. This creates a drain of energy and therefore resources from the body. This vortex is relative to issues of relationships, creativity, and self-expression. There is inflammation in the area as well as debris, crystallized energy that acts as an irritant in the system. We dissipate the inflammation and remove and transmute the debris into normal light frequencies. Next we decompress a dense deep blockage around the rim of the base of this vortex. We extract the vortex from within the body and clarify it of all stagnant energy. Next we correct polarities and return it to its normal upright presentation. Next we root the vortex firmly in place and calibrate for correction of oscillation and density. We attune the vortex to within normal limits of this area.

The second vortex is torn and leaking energy. We assimilate and repair this vortex. Next we calibrate to correct shape and density and attune to correction and enhancement of frequency sets. Further, we root the vortex in perfect position.

The first vortex is not functioning. We correct placement on plane, angulation, and frequency relationships until it becomes fully functional once again.

The emotional body is corded to the physical and mental bodies. It is swollen in self-protection. This being does not receive enough nurturing, especially from self. We suggest that she share with herself those things which bring comfort and fullness into her heart so that her emotional being becomes of greater healthfulness. We remove and destroy the cordings from all three bodies and calibrate the emotional body to normalization of size and density. Next we dissipate the moderate and dense blockages that we have found within this body and attune the body to uniformity and perfection.

The mental body is angulated 45 degrees off plane to the west. We correct positioning.

The causal bodies are off plane center and parallel. We correct their positioning.

The body of this soul is perfect as it would be. The area around this body is riddled with small, moderate and severe cylindrical blockages. These are Karmic instances that are at play or have not been satisfied. We are given that self-empowerment has been a many lifetime struggle for this being as well as the ability to connect deeply with others because of her fears. We decompress the *blockages in order that this soul can see past her challenges and to learn from and resolve them if she chooses. We clarify this field to uniformity and repair the field of all injury. This does not remove Karma, simply allows for the soul to experience more astutely and clearly.*

The body of this being is swollen in a mirrored fashion to what was noted in the emotional body. The physical reaction is a response to the emotional energies. We lay in a vector of reprogramming energy that will long term reinstruct the physicality toward a more desirable and healthful expression of self.

One would do well to embrace love, the love of self first and then for others without the fear of loss. She would realize that in this now she is safe, she has everything that she needs, and it is only her fear that keeps some of those things from becoming tangible experiences for her. Changing this experience only requires changing perception of self. She must want to have her life in order to have it. She must feel valid in order to be valid She must realize her perfection in order to experience it. Of course she is all that and more, yet denies these things in deference to others who led her to believe differently. That belief is untruth. She is magnificent.

End of session.

Exercise Seven: Learning to Work Long Distance

Long distance connections are already within us, we just need to realize that and have no doubt as to their validity. A friend of mine, Joseph Crane, and his mentor, Alexander Everett (now deceased from this world), came up with a terrific exercise that you can do to open your long distance awareness. This exercise works best when shared by two or more people who are working together. With Joe's permission, here is the exercise:

Following this description there is an outline of a body. It is neither male nor female so can apply to anyone. Make copies of the body on separate sheets of paper so that you can write on them.

Continued

With your friend or friends, take a 3˝ × 5˝ card and

* *Think of someone you know who has an illness or serious life problems.*

* *Write their first name on the top of the card. Do not use their full name.*

* *Under the person's first name, describe everything about the person such as their hair color, eyes, complexion, general build, height, and any distinguishing features such as big nose, pointy chin, salt and pepper hair. In other words, lots of detail so another person would recognize them by sight if they walked into the room. Do not write what the problems or illness are!*

* *Put your name on the back of the card.*

* *Once you are finished, exchange cards with your friends. Make sure they don't know the person you described or get their own card back.*

* *Now it is time to address the paper that you have with the image of the blank body. Take the description of the person on the card, and imagine that the body on the paper is that person.*

* *Close your eyes and place your hands on or over the paper body, and using your intuition, imagine that you are feeling the body of the person who is described on your card. Use your third eye and all of your senses.*

* *Construct a perfect body in your mind from the skeleton outward to compare against that body on the paper.*

* *Use your hand or hands and lightly allow them to move across the body. What do you feel? Are there warm or cold areas? Do different areas of the body give you feelings, emotions, sensations, or even specific or general information about that person? If so, make a note on the paper next to that part of the body. Don't get stuck in too much detail; just write enough so you can remember your impression later. Are there bumps on the paper, rough areas, sticky areas, and do*

those have any information about the body? Do you sense anything about this person that isn't physical?

- When you are finished, ask the body if there is anything else it would like to share with you. If you have any immediate impressions after asking that question, write those down.

- When everyone is finished, take turns sharing what you have found on your paper body. Ask the person who provided their description to validate whether or not your impressions are similar to what the live person is experiencing.

What you will find as you discuss your impressions in relation to the actual information provided by your friends is that you already know how to "tap in"; you just didn't realize it. I am always awed by the accuracy of my students when they do this exercise . . . and so are they!

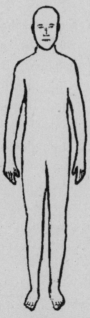

Body for Long Distance Exercise
©Meg Blackburn Losey and Spirit Light Resources 2001.

The End Is Only the Beginning

Healing with our Seventh Sense isn't just a process; it is the creation of life, of healing, of the infinite possibilities that are available to our clients and us. It is a mergence between our infinite soul and those of others. Simply put, healing with our Seventh Sense brings forward the powers of creation in such potent ways that miracles can and do happen.

What I have shared in this book is only the beginning of what is possible when we step aside from our limited human perceptions and are willing to leap beyond our local reality and into infinite worlds beyond our complete understanding. We can never logically understand most of what happens beyond our five senses because it isn't logical. Instead, all else is part of our intricately woven tapestry within a greater one.

When we become competent with working within these vast layers of truth, we become able to command new and different realities. We are mechanisms of creation. We are the impetus of change. We are the consciousness within the living One.

It is easy to doubt what we can't see or feel or touch, but that doesn't make any of it less real or effective. Our willingness to become unconditional as living aspects of our source allows us to open doors that some have known about from the before times and throughout countless millennia. To us, some of these ideas and practices seem new, but they are not. They are cryptically written about in ancient texts, and they have been practiced quietly in temples as secret rites and in back rooms, hidden from the general public, and considered to be only esoteric in nature. To me, healing such as this goes far beyond the body mind spirit connections and into realms of the most basic forms of being. We are eternity contained within bodies that feel, sense, know, and fear. We dream we laugh we cry we hope we love and we are, in our perceptions complexity expressed in biological form. But what if now we began to realize that to touch the light is to become the very Creator that we pray to?

What if we became able to understand who we really are and what we can do? What if we found the faith to know that miracles are not something that happen only by the actions of those we hold sacred, but can be brought forth by us as humanity who have chosen to express our parts of the living One? What then?

The possibilities are endless. They are only restricted by our unwillingness to step out of our comfortable known realities.

All it takes to change those perceptions is to step back into our innocence, to allow ourselves to be in awe, to have immutable faith, to have the courage to become immersed into the unknown and to act solely from our hearts, from a pure state of love, from *our* sacred being. We are that.

It is my deepest desire that the tools that I have provided in this book will propagate into this world as keys to greater being. Sometimes just knowing is enough to change our lives. Sometimes we need to apply our tools practically to completely comprehend what we can do, but always we need to believe that there are powers greater than we can ever understand and that they are at our finger-tips. All we need to do is say yes.

SUGGESTED READING

Brennan, Barbara. *Hands of Light: A Guide to Healing Through the Human Energy Field.* New York: Bantam, 1988.

Clark, Hulda Regehr. *The Cure for All Diseases.*, 1995 Chula Vista CA: New Century Press, 1995.

Dale, Cyndi. *The Subtle Body: An Encyclopedia of Your Energetic Anatomy.* Sounds True, Incorporated, 2009.

Einstein, Albert, and Greene, Brian. *The Meaning of Relativity, Fifth Ed.: Including the Relativistic Theory of the Non-Symmetric Field.* Princeton NJ: Princeton Science Library, 2004.

Greene, Brian. *The Expanse of Reality: Parallel Universes and the Search for the Deep Laws of the Cosmos.* New York: Alfred Knopf., 2011.

Greene, Brian. *The Elegant Universe: Superstrings, Hidden Dimensions, and the Quest for the Ultimate Theory.*) New York: Vintage Books, 2000.

Greene, Brian. *The Fabric of the Cosmos: Space, Time, and the Texture of Reality.* New York: Vintage, 2005.

Haley, Daniel. *Politics in Healing: The Suppression and Manipulation of American Medicine.* Washington DC: Potomac Valley Press, 2000.

Hawking, Steven. *The Grand Design.* New York: Bantam, 2010.

Lipton, Bruce. *The Biology of Belief: Unleashing the Power of Consciousness, Matter, and Miracles.* Carlsbad, CA: Hay House, 2008.

Losey, Meg Blackburn; *The Secret History of Consciousness.* , San Francisco: Red Wheel Weiser, 2010.

McTaggart, Lynne. *The Field: The Quest for the Secret Force of the Universe.* New York: Harper Paperbacks, 2008.

McTaggart, Lynne. *The Intention Experiment: Using Your Thoughts to Change Your Life and the World.* New York: Free Press, 2008.

Pert, Candace. *Molecules of Emotion: The Science Behind Mind–Body Medicine, 1st Ed.* New York: Simon & Schuster, 1999.

Peirce, Penney. *Frequency: The Power of Personal Vibration.* New York: Atria Books/Beyond Words, 2009.

Peirce, Penney. *The Intuitive Way: The Definitive Guide to Increasing Your Awareness, 1st Ed.* Atria Books/Beyond Words, 2009.

Talbot, Michael. *The Holographic Universe.* New York: HarperCollins, 1992.

Talbot, Michael. *Mysticism and the New Physics. (Compass)* New York: Penguin, 1993.

Tolle, Eckhart. *The Power of Now: A Guide to Spiritual Enlightenment.* Novato, CA: New World Library, 2004

ABOUT THE AUTHOR

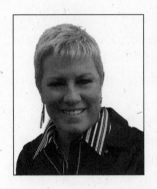

Meg Blackburn, PhD, is the host of "Cosmic Particles" internet radio show. She is the author of the bestselling *The Secret History of Consciousness, Parenting the Children of Now, Conversations with the Children of Now,* the international bestseller *The Children of Now, Crystalline Children, Indigo Children, Star Kids, Angels on Earth and The Phenomenon of Transitional Children, Pyramids of Light, Awakening to Multi-dimensional Reality,* and the *Online Messages.* She is also a contributor to *The Mystery of 2012* anthology and a regular contributor in many magazines and other publications.

TO OUR READERS